KUNDALINI YOGA

The Flow of

Eternal Power

An Easy Guide to the Yoga of Awareness
As taught by Yogi Bhajan, Ph.D.

SHAKTI PARWHA KAUR KHALSA

Time Capsule Books
P.O. Box 351149
Los Angeles, California 90035

FIRST EDITION
Copyright © 1996 Shakti Parwha Kaur Khalsa
Los Angeles, California

First Printing, June 1996
Second Printing, January 1997

ISBN 0-9639847-6-4
Library of Congress Catalog Card Number: 96-85357

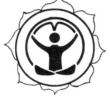

APPROVED BY THE KUNDALINI RESEARCH INSTITUTE
This book has received the KRI seal of approval which
is granted only to those products which have been
approved through the Kundalini Research Institute
review process for the accuracy and integrity of those
portions which embody the technology of Kundalini
Yoga and 3HO lifestyle as taught by Yogi Bhajan.

Thanks to 3HO Foundation for permission to use previously published material.

PRINTED IN CANADA

Distributed by
Ancient Healing Ways
Route 3, Box 259
Espanola, New Mexico 87532
(800) 359-2940

DEDICATION

This book is dedicated to those who have
loved me, my best Teachers:

My Mother,
who taught me to smile
and gave me unshakable faith in God.

My Two Brothers,
who showed me that men can be
kind and wonderful.

Yogi Bhajan, my Spiritual Teacher,
who gave me my Self.

His life of infinite compassion,
inexhaustible patience
and constant sacrifice
has provided an awesome example of

Keeping Up!

DESIGN & LAYOUT
Guru Raj Kaur Khalsa

FRONT COVER ART & DESIGN
Seva Kaur Khalsa

COVER PRODUCTION & DESIGN
Pritpal Singh Khalsa

ILLUSTRATIONS
Shabad Kaur Khalsa

ILLUSTRATIVE CONSULTANT
Shiva Singh Khalsa

PRINTING
Hari Nam Singh Khalsa
GRD Graphic Services, 416-929-8018
Toronto, Ontario, Canada

YOGA POSTURES

Photographs
Sat Simran Kaur Khalsa
Peraim Kaur Khalsa

Demonstrated by
Sadhana Kaur Khalsa
Siri Simran Kaur Khalsa
Nam Kaur Khalsa

BACK COVER PHOTOGRAPH
Sardarni Guru Amrit Kaur Khalsa

Acknowledgements

One of the pillars of my faith is called *seva*. It means "selfless service." The spirit of *seva* permeated the creation of this book. Many wonderful people gave generously of their expertise, time, and energy during the four and a half years it took to complete. I had made three earlier attempts to write this book several years before the crucial December, 1991, Khalsa Council workshop facilitated by Subagh Singh Khalsa that motivated me to focus and commit to completing it. Guruka Singh Khalsa and Siri Ved Kaur Khalsa gave valuable editorial input to those earlier versions.

Dr. Sat Kaur Khalsa shared with me three useful—and for me imperative—suggestions. If you're planning to write a book, I suggest you also follow them. They worked for me! 1) Make appointments with yourself for the actual time you plan to work on the book, write them down, and honor them. Start at the time you're committed to, and stop at the time you predetermined. Then write down your next appointment and stick to it. 2) Chant and pray before each writing session. 3) Just write, before you try to edit. Get the whole thing down on paper (or in the computer) before you start the editing process. Writing and editing are two different modes.

In the proofreading and editing department I had extremely useful comments from my designated readers, Harijot Kaur Khalsa, Sat Narayan Simran Kaur, Shanti Kaur Khalsa, Susan Liebman Ladd, and Ted Garon. (Harijot's artistic eye also helped in selecting the illustrations.) Gobind Kaur Khalsa not only held up under the marathon final proofreading sessions to meet the printer's deadline, but in the early stages helped organize the chapters. Gurupreet Kaur Khalsa jumped in at a moment's notice to proofread, as did Ek Ong Kar Kaur Khalsa, and Sahib Amar Kaur Khalsa, computer expert, volunteered to enter all the punctuation and spelling corrections needed on the first draft.

Both Sat Simran Kaur Khalsa and Peraim Kaur Khalsa spent endless hours trying to take just the right photos to illustrate the yoga postures. Nam Kaur Khalsa, Siri Simran Kaur Khalsa, and Sadhana Kaur Khalsa demonstrated not only great yogic flexibility, but patience and endurance. A special salute to Sardarni Guru Amrit Kaur who was able to perform the miracle of taking a usable photo of me.

Thanks to Guru Raj Kaur Khalsa and Shabad Kaur Khalsa who really served above and beyond the call of duty!

My deepest gratitude to all of the above, as well as to Aradhana Singh Khalsa, Dr. Gurucharan Singh Khalsa, Hari Nam Singh Khalsa, Jagat Joti Singh Khalsa, and the scores of others who have given such enthusiastic encouragement and support to this project. God bless you each and all. Your kindness is engraved in my heart.

Sat Nam.

Foreword

Where to Begin? First steps are important and often color the rest of the journey. This book puts you on secure footing in the right direction for a more fulfilled life and an awakened consciousness.

Shakti's style to mix profound ideas with humor and a personal almost "chatty" conversation makes the journey fun and painless. She constantly helps you along with a song, a poem, a story, and just enough bullet points to insure you remember what's important.

A student who had studied for many years had become confused with all the opinions and the hundreds of approaches. All the student wanted was clear guidance to establish a personal practice for a happy and spirit filled life. The student approached a master yogi. The yogi smiled and spread his fingers. He placed the little finger at the navel and the thumb tip at the heart. He said, "The journey you must travel is only six inches long. Begin at the navel and reach the heart."

In other words, all the studies and intellectual ideas are best dealt with by a practice, a way of living that takes you from the concerns of control and survival to the experience of the heart, connected and free. The Kundalini energy of awareness is initiated in the body from the navel. Self understanding awakens in the heart center.

The master said a lot with a simple gesture.

This is Shakti's special gift. From her first chapter to the last you travel from basic habits to the heart center of living a better life with a truer sense of your self.

I am biased. I learned Kundalini Yoga at the feet of Yogi Bhajan and from Shakti Parwha in 1969. I have trained teachers of this science as Director of Training for Kundalini Research Institute and 3HO for over twenty years. In all this time I have not found a better place to start than with the wit and wisdom of Shakti.

I am grateful for her clarity, fidelity to the original teachings, and her decades of service to share this with all.

Enjoy one of the best and quickest introductions to this sacred science of being human.

MSS Gurucharan Singh Khalsa, Ph. D.
Director of Training KRI
(Kundalini Research Institute)

Contents

Section Two
THINGS TO DO

Section One

THINGS TO KNOW

and a Few Things to Try

Before You Begin . . .

Always consult your physician before beginning this or any other exercise program. Nothing in this book is to be construed as medical advice. The benefits attributed to the practice of Kundalini Yoga come from the centuries-old yogic tradition. Results will vary with individuals.

You Are Here ☞

How to Read This Book

This book is brazenly personal. I have taken the marvelous technology of Kundalini Yoga as taught by my spiritual teacher, Yogi Bhajan, the Master of Kundalini Yoga, and presented it in my own conversational style. This is the way I have been teaching students in Kundalini Yoga Beginners classes for twenty-seven years: straight, simple, and with a smile!

This is not a manual or a textbook but it does have specific "things" you can do: breathing, stretching, chanting, meditating. I've also included some psychological, philosophical, and I hope, inspirational commentary, plus many excerpts from Yogi Bhajan's lectures. There are some personal anecdotes and a sprinkling of my own poetry. Each topic could be a whole book in itself. Believe it or not, I've tried to be brief, but it's difficult to be brief and thorough at the same time.

You'll find new ideas, new ways of looking at yourself and the people in your life, plus some yogic tidbits that you can apply to everyday activities. I want this book to whet your appetite to experience more of the vast technology of Kundalini Yoga. I know it can transform your life from the inside out and the outside in. I know, because I tried it. You won't know until *you* try it. You will find most quotes in this book are Yogi Bhajan's words. After all, he's the Master Yogi! Here is the first:

"Doing is Believing."

I genuinely love and value the teachings I'm about to share with you. I want as many people as possible to benefit from them because I know that the

1

more people who practice Kundalini Yoga, the more happy people there will be in the world. The more happy people there are in the world, the better the world is going to be for me to live in!

I hope you'll read this book with an open mind and an open heart, and practice the exercises and meditations. They have transformed my life; I know they can do the same for you.

You don't have to read this book in exact order (though it's preferable) but I do recommend that after you finish this that you read the first five chapters in sequence. They will get you off to a good start. Then, if you wish, you can go to the Table of Contents, see what grabs you, and read that next. The book is organized into two sections: the first part is *Things To Know* (and a few things to try) and the second part is specific *Things To Do*.

Starting right now, you CAN change your life. You CAN be Bountiful, Blissful & Beautiful. In fact, you already are! You just have to experience it.

This can't be a step-by-step book, because it's a book about life and we live life on many different levels going in many different directions all at the same time. We have a physical life, a mental life, and a spiritual life happening simultaneously. These pages contain a blueprint for building a healthy, happy, and holy life. Yogi Bhajan calls it the "3HO way of life." *It is your birthright*. This concept was one of the first things Yogi Bhajan talked about when I met him in 1968. The 3HO Foundation was born as a result of his inspiration. Now a world-wide organization with 300 centers in thirty-five countries, 3HO is dedicated to sharing these life affirming teachings.

I have to pause here and explain what I mean by "holy," otherwise you may get the wrong impression. Holy does NOT mean to be "holier than thou." It does not mean to be sanctimonious. The 3HO yogic definition of holy is pretty straightforward. It has two parts: First, "Do unto others what you want them to do unto you" (sound familiar?), and second, "Receive each inhalation consciously, gratefully aware that each breath you receive is a gift!"

2

Learning how the yogis define concepts gives us a welcome new perspective on life. That's another feature of this book, getting a new perspective on everything, including who you are.

I refuse to claim that reading this book and learning new terms will solve all your problems. But it will give you powerful, practical tools to meet the challenges in your life and consciously, courageously conquer them.

Starting right now, you *can* change your life! As Yogi Bhajan says, "you *can* be: Bountiful, Blissful, and Beautiful. In fact, you ALREADY ARE! You just have to experience it.

Rx

For best digestion: Take a few chapters at a time; read slowly and chew thoroughly. Repeat as often as necessary.
No. of Refills: Unlimited
Exp. Date: none

1

What's It All About?

You Don't Have to Be a Pretzel

Yogi Bhajan pointed to me and said to the class he was teaching at Claremont College, "See, Shakti's doing it; if she can do it, anybody can do it."

That was in 1969. I still consider myself one of the least physically coordinated people on the planet, and yet, here I am, twenty-seven years later, not only doing Kundalini Yoga, but teaching it, and writing a book about it, because I sincerely believe it's true, if I can do it, anybody can!

The physical exercise part of Kundalini Yoga is just one aspect of this Yoga of Awareness. Among the many outrageous quotes from Yogi Bhajan is, "If flexibility of the body is the only yoga, then clowns in the circus are the best yogis." Important as the physical body is, and as desirable as flexibility is, there is much more to be gained from yoga, there is your entire happiness and success in life.

When you buy a new automobile, a toaster, or a VCR (almost anything with moving parts) the manufacturer provides a book of instructions. The owner's manual recommends procedures to get maximum efficiency. It lists checkpoints and times for periodic maintenance. It tells you what to look for if it's not working properly and it suggests how to avoid future problems.

So where are the instructions for your care and maintenance? When you were born you didn't come neatly packaged with a tag tied around your big toe, labeled "Care and Feeding." Though a human being is surely one of the most complicated mechanisms ever created, still an instruction manual isn't provided with each newborn baby. Perhaps the Manufacturer assumed that mothers would study directly with the experts to learn how to care for the new arrival. And who are these "experts"? Not the psychologists and pediatricians, not well-meaning friends and neighbors,

5

mothers and grandmothers (though the latter probably have learned a lot through trial and error).

The trained experts, the people who developed the finest methods to care for, maintain, and get maximum mileage out of this human mechanism (not just physically, but mentally, emotionally, and spiritually), were the yogis.

Detailed information on the care and feeding, maintenance and preservation of a human being was revealed to the yogis thousands of years ago. They have been custodians of this technology ever since. They are the expert mechanics, scientists, engineers, and problem-solvers for the intricate human machine in all its aspects: body, mind, and soul.

THE SCIENCE OF KUNDALINI YOGA

For thousands of years this yogic knowledge was carefully handed down by oral tradition from Master to disciple. The Master spoke, the student memorized and practiced. Eventually a portion of this vast body of knowledge leading to enlightenment, or self-mastery, was written down. Some of these sacred teachings can be found in ancient Vedic texts.[1]

There's a yogic art and science to all aspects of human life. There's a yogic way to get up in the morning; there's a yogic way to go to sleep at night. A way to eat, and a way to breathe! Virtually every aspect of human existence has an enlightened, efficient, and effective way to do it. This legacy of technical and spiritual knowledge that Yogi Bhajan studied and mastered in India is the gift he brought to the West.

THE YOGI'S GIFT

Kundalini Yoga was always kept very secret. It was never taught publicly until 1969, when Yogi Bhajan challenged the ages-old tradition of secrecy.

He spent many years in India learning, mastering, and perfecting the habits and practices of Kundalini Yoga. It sometimes took months of waiting patiently and being tested in many ways before a Teacher would reveal anything at all to him. Yet he has offered to share these ancient secrets with us, openly and honestly. His motive? Compassion. He wants us to stop suffering. He sees the reality of our inner beauty, power, and potential and he wants us to discover it for ourselves.

Yogi Bhajan started teaching Kundalini Yoga in easy-to-digest yogic "tid-bits." I want to share these teachings with you that same way. I want to make it as simple and easy as I can for you to apply them in your daily life so you can feel better, look better, and be a happier person.

Of all the technology and wisdom that Yogi Bhajan could have taught from his vast storehouse of mastery, he chose to teach Kundalini Yoga

It is the birthright of every human being to be healthy, happy and holy.

because it is so effective, comprehensive, and "do-able."

This is a yoga for householders, for people who have to cope with the daily challenges and stresses of holding jobs, raising families, managing businesses. It gives results in the shortest possible time. It does not require you to leave your home, become an ascetic or sit in a cave. Kundalini Yoga is for everyone who wants the skills to cope successfully with the challenges of living in this day and age.[2] (And you don't have to be a pretzel. For the physical exercises, if you can breathe, and just lean in the right direction, you'll be benefitted. I told you, if I can do it, anybody can.)

WHAT DOES KUNDALINI YOGA DO?

The practice of Kundalini Yoga balances the glandular system, strengthens the nervous system and enables us to harness the energy of the mind and the emotions, so we can be in control of ourselves, rather than being controlled by our thoughts and feelings.

Another purpose of this book is to dispel the mystery, the myths and misunderstanding, that exist about Kundalini Yoga. It is a precious gem of sacred knowledge and power. I am going to show you some of its many brilliant facets. It can make your life shine. It is like a magic jewel that I can give to you and still keep for myself. In fact, sharing it makes it brighter for me!

THE GOAL

Kundalini Yoga is designed to give you "hands on" experience of your highest consciousness. It teaches a method by which you can achieve the sacred purpose of your life. This can be described in many ways, such as:

7

- Experience your inner light of consciousness.
- Experience your own highest consciousness.
- Discover your real Identity.

The practices enable you to merge with or "yoke" with the universal Self. This merging of individual consciousness with universal consciousness creates a "divine union" called "yoga."

The practice that leads to this state of self-mastery is also called "yoga." So the road and the destination have the same name, "yoga." There are many different kinds, or schools of yoga. *(See Many Paths.)* Those who practice yoga are called yogis and those who master yoga are also called yogis.

The technology of Kundalini Yoga applies its science to our bodies and minds, and is aimed at spirit which has no boundaries, no discrimination. Therefore it is for everyone. It is universal and nondenominational.

IS YOGA A RELIGION?

Kundalini Yoga is not a religion. Kundalini Yoga is a Sacred Science. It is sacred because it deals with the GOD ("G": that which Generates; "O": that which Organizes; "D": that which Delivers or Destroys) in you. It is scientific because it provides a technology, a method by which anyone who practices it can experience that divine identity within. The way you choose to worship that G-O-D is your religion.

Yes, Kundalini Yoga does require FAITH (not belief), just as a course in chemistry requires the faith of the student to do the laboratory experiments so he can prove the validity of the formulas for himself.

LONG TERM GAIN / SHORT TERM GAIN

As you work toward achieving the goal of Yoga or liberation, you become more capable, more confident, and more efficient in whatever you're doing in your external life. Simultaneously, you become progressively more aware of yourself on all levels. It's a win/win situation!

SECRETS OF POWER

To fully appreciate the value of this great gift Yogi Bhajan has brought us, we need to understand why, for thousands of years, the Yogis kept it secret. They preserved and carefully guarded the knowledge of the inner and outer workings of a human being, very cautiously revealing the technology, selectively passing it down verbally from Master to chosen disciple. They were selective because knowledge gives power, and power can corrupt. Traditionally, disciples had to spend many years proving their trustworthiness and ethical purity to receive the sacred science of Kundalini Yoga. Only after the student demonstrated humility, self-discipline, and obedience would the Teacher reveal the secret Kriyas. Yet Yogi Bhajan has taken it upon himself to share his knowledge openly with everyone. *(See the chapter My Spiritual Teacher for more about this remarkable human being, Master of Kundalini Yoga and White Tantric Yoga.)* He has done this in order to prepare humanity for the major changes that the planet is going through. The world we knew even ten years ago has totally changed—geographically, socially, economically, morally. We have already crossed from the Piscean Age into the Age of Aquarius.[3] As he has said, "What used to work, won't work anymore." It's a new Age already, and this ancient technology of Kundalini Yoga can give us the awareness and the strength to make our transition smoother.

THE POWER OF PRANA

Kundalini Yoga deals specifically with the most powerful thing in the universe, the basic life energy, prana. Prana is the sub-atomic energy, the life force. It was known to yogis for thousands of years, long before the scientists split the atom. It is prana that you receive with every breath. It's mighty powerful stuff. Kundalini Yoga is the path of discovery of the source of the prana in us and teaches us how to use it.

WHY PRACTICE KUNDALINI YOGA?

People decide to practice Kundalini Yoga for many reasons. Possibly your chiropractor suggested it. Or your psychologist, physician, or next-door neighbor recommended it to help you relax, cope with stress, and find peace of mind. Or, perhaps you're simply curious. It doesn't matter what your reason, you

9

are welcome! But be warned: If you genuinely practice it, you will find yourself and your life changing. If you don't want to change, if you're totally content with yourself and your life as it is now, then don't go any further. But if you want to explore the possibilities of your highest potential, then keep reading.

Kundalini Yoga is much more than just a system of physical exercises. It is a dynamic, powerful tool for expanding awareness. Approach it with respect, with reverence, and with openness.

The purpose of this book is to get you to try it for yourself, so you can have your own experience of the benefits it has to offer.

"DOING IS BELIEVING."

Let the words on these pages help you take the next step on your personal journey of self-discovery. You are, indeed, a unique and wonderful being with a very special destiny. Let Kundalini Yoga, the Yoga of Awareness, help you achieve your personal best!

2
One Goal

Spiritual Travel

All things come from God, everything will eventually return to God, including you. How you get there is your particular path. The Yogi wants to have that experience sooner and chooses a path to travel that best suits his[1] temperament and capabilities.

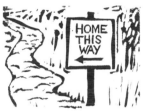

Different paths suit different people. Going for a hike? You can make the rugged, uphill climb or follow well-marked trails and stroll along at a leisurely pace. Want to go farther? You can fly direct to New York from Los Angeles, or make stops along the way. You can even change planes. If you have lots of time, you may decide to take a bus or a train along the scenic route. Some folks enjoy driving across country. The choice of "how" to get there is yours. The choice of "when" to get there is affected by the "how." The "where" is predetermined, because although there are many paths back "Home," there's no place else to go.

Kundalini Yoga might be called the direct, non-stop jet route. It is a very comprehensive technology, yet ideally suited to people who lead active lives in today's world.

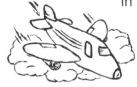

In the back of this book you can read brief descriptions of some of the other paths of yoga. Since Kundalini Yoga is what this book is all about, I'm going to give it a lot more space than the others. I think that's fair, don't you?

Kundalini Yoga balances the glandular system, strengthens the 72,000 nerves in the body, expands the lung capacity, and purifies the bloodstream. It brings balance to the body, mind, and soul. It teaches   positive, self-

[1] Anytime you see "he" or "his" for a non-specific person, please assume I also include "she" and "her." Let's save ink.

11

WHAT DOES "YOGA" MEAN?

"What does yoga mean? Yoga means to be united. When you unite with your soul and unite with the One who gave you the soul, that's what yoga is. Do it in a royal way, it's called Raj Yoga. Do it in a graceful way, then it's called Karma Yoga, Bhakti Yoga, Shakti Yoga... When you do it in an absolutely involved conscious way and you put your involved consciousness on the top of it, they call it Kundalini Yoga— uncoil yourself. You reveal yourself, you identify yourself. That is called Kundalini Yoga and Sikhs call it SAT NAM..."

—Yogi Bhajan, Nov. 30, 1988

"Kundalini Yoga is the science to unite the finite with Infinity and it's the art to experience Infinity in the finite. All those people who practice Kundalini Yoga don't have to have different definitions. This is it. It is straight. It is simple. It creates no complications."

—Yogi Bhajan, Oct. 27, 1988

"What is the Kundalini? The creative potential of the man."

—Teachings of Yogi Bhajan, p. 177

empowering attitudes of thinking. It is on-the-job-training for success and excellence in life. It builds inner strength and self awareness so you can fulfill your highest potential.

In Kundalini Yoga we harness the mental, physical, and nervous energies of the body and put them under the domain of the will, which is the instrument of the soul. Kundalini Yoga perfects the finite life while connecting it to the Infinite experience.

3

Ong Namo Guru Dev Namo

Tuning In

We *always* tune in before doing any practice of Kundalini Yoga.

When you want to watch your favorite television show, you have to select the right channel. If you want to watch the World Series, you don't turn to the Home-Shopping channel. You get what you want by selecting the particular wavelength that is broadcasting the program you want to see.

The T.V. log has dozens of listings. All the T.V. stations broadcast simultaneously. Your screen shows only the particular one you have selected. Why? Because of the principle of attunement. You get the station or channel you want by tuning to the correct frequency. When you use the right "call letters" you get the channel you want. This same principle governs the science of mantra.

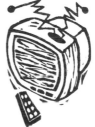

Tuning in is simply changing channels on the television of your mind.

MANTRA

We live in a sea of energy. Energy vibrates. There's a particular vibratory frequency corresponding to every sound in the universe. By vibrating a particular combination of sounds (syllables), you tune-in to various levels of intelligence or consciousness. You're choosing programs all the time, whether you know it or not.

Consciously or unconsciously, purposely or at random, you personally choose the programs that play on the screen of your mind by the thoughts you think (vibrate) and the words you speak (vibrate).

Mantras are combinations of syllables consciously constructed to connect with specific levels of intelligence. Using a mantra is like dialing a phone number. If you want to talk with your friend in Florida, you don't call the San Diego Zoo.

The knowledge of the meaning and power of sounds and the use of the sound current is contained in the ancient technology of Mantra Yoga. It is a major factor in the practice of Kundalini Yoga.

Spirituality cannot be taught, it has to be caught, like the measles.

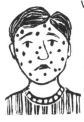

We've already said that Kundalini Yoga is a sacred science. It is a spiritual practice. "Spirituality" is contagious. You have to get it from someone who's got it. That's why we start each class by "tuning in" to the wavelength of the teachers who've "got it"—so we can receive their vibration. The mantra we use to accomplish this is **ONG NAMO GURU DEV NAMO**. These code letters not only invoke the blessing of your own highest self, but they open the protective link between you and the long line of Spiritual Masters who have preceded us on the path. This transmitting of higher consciousness from Master to disciple which has been going on for thousands of years is sometimes called the "golden chain." Yogi Bhajan, Master of Kundalini Yoga, is the immediate connection to this chain for all of us who practice Kundalini Yoga.

ONG NAMO GURU DEV NAMO is chanted (vibrated) to assure the purest inner guidance for your practice of Kundalini Yoga.

Here's how to turn the dial of your mind and switch to the channel that will give you the clearest reception for the technology of Kundalini Yoga, and the elevated consciousness (vibration) that comes with it. I'm going to explain this in great detail, because it's really important that you get started correctly from the very beginning.

Ready? Get set:

Sit with your spine straight. Preferably sit cross-legged on the floor (use a mat, folded blanket, or something firm for padding). In yogic terms, this cross-legged position is called Sukh Asan which translates as "easy-pose," though it may not be easy for you. If you can't sit on the floor, you can sit on a chair, just make sure that both feet are planted firmly on the floor with weight equally balanced. Keep your spine straight. Place the palms of your hands flat together at the center of your chest, fingers pointing upward at a very slight angle outward. The sides of your thumbs press lightly but firmly at the center of the sternum. This pressure stimulates a nerve ending that goes up to the brain; we call it the "mind nerve." This mudra (hand position) is called "Prayer Pose." Not only does it make you look saintly (not a bad image), but it helps concentration. Being able to concentrate, being one-pointed, and able to keep your attention focused is not only useful for meditation; it also comes in handy for baking a cake, writing a symphony, or riding a bicycle. Successful completion of any job requires us to corral and harness the multitude of scattered thought fragments flying wildly about in our untrained minds.

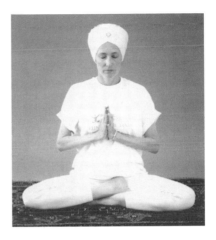

Prayer Pose in
Sukh Asan
(Easy Pose)

Keep the palms pressed firmly together. The palms contain nerve endings corresponding to the left and right hemispheres of the brain. Pressing them together helps to balance the logical hemisphere of the brain with the creative, intuitive hemisphere. This balance is important for successful concentration.

Pull your chin back slightly, to help straighten the spine, allowing freer movement of the Kundalini energy upwards.

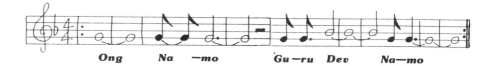

Ong　　Na　—mo　　　'Gu—ru　Dev　　Na—mo

ONG NAMO GURU DEV NAMO

"I Bow to the Creator, to the Divine Teacher Within."

- **ONG** means the Creator - the One Who created you.
- **NAMO** means reverent greetings, salutations.
- **GURU** is the giver of the technology, the Teacher.
    Teacher: the one who gets rid of ignorance
    GU = darkness, **RU** = light, that which dispels darkness.
- **DEV** means transparent (nonphysical).

Ready? Read the following instructions first, then close your eyes, keeping them focused at the center of your forehead and begin.

Take several long deep breaths, inhaling deeply through your nose, then exhaling completely out through the nose. Do this several times, then:

Inhale deeply through the nose, and vibrate the syllable **ONG** at the back of the throat and feel the sound going out through the nose.

Then slide into the sound **NAMO** (the NA is a short syllable, while the MO is extended. *See pronunciation guide.*) and complete the rest of the mantra, raising the pitch of the syllable **DEV** (which rhymes with "save") about a third-tone higher than the rest of the mantra.

Finish exhaling all the breath as you chant the final **NAMO**.

If you can do it, chant the entire mantra all in one breath without a pause. If you find you need to catch your breath slightly before chanting **G'ROO** (rhymes with "who"), you can take a quick sip of air through the mouth after Ong Namo, just as you do automatically when you are speaking, but don't inhale through the nose during the mantra. (Note, the syllable GU in Guru, is extremely brief.)

After each complete round, inhale very deeply through the nose before you chant the entire mantra again. Continue this sequence at least three times, breathing only through the nose. Continue chanting **ONG NAMO GURU DEV NAMO** as many more times as you wish until you feel "connected." It is like letting the phone ring until someone picks up.

There is a basic melody we usually use, but the melody is not so important as the rhythm and the breath. This holds true for all mantras — the most important factors are the rhythm and the breath.

When you have finished chanting **ONG NAMO GURU DEV NAMO**, inhale deeply. Feel yourself being filled with energy, life, light and joy! Hold the breath as long as you can do so comfortably. Then exhale completely, feeling the breath carrying away tension and fatigue. Feel yourself getting rid of worry or disease. Take a few more of these long deep breaths, using each breath as a self-healing meditation. There are many powerful meditations, but there is nothing more powerful than meditation on the breath.

Let me repeat: Always remember to chant **ONG NAMO GURU DEV NAMO** at least three times before you begin each session of Kundalini Yoga. Be conscious of the important meaning of the mantra while you are chanting so that it does not become a mere ritual.

ONG NAMO GURU DEV NAMO is such a valuable mantra that Yogi Bhajan had a forty-five minute tape of it made with continuous chanting by Nirinjan Kaur. We often meditate or chant along with it during yoga classes, and it's used frequently for meditation in White Tantric Yoga video courses. The beautiful melody on this tape is different from the original.

> **IMPORTANT CONCEPTS:**
>
> 1. There is nothing more powerful than meditation on your breath.
>
> 2. Chanting is not singing. It is not speaking. It is vibrating.
>
> 3. To make any mantra more effective, chant from your navel point.

4

Breath of Life

HOW TO BREATHE (DON'T I ALREADY KNOW HOW?)
We give our children piano lessons, we eagerly encourage them to walk and talk, but how many of us train them to breathe? Did your parents teach you? The good news is that we are born with enough built-in breathing skill to keep us alive. The bad news is that until we learn to breathe consciously, we're only "half-alive." We're like champion racing cars that never get out of first gear.

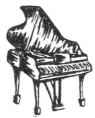

INSPIRATION—ASPIRATION: RESPIRATION !

Some of the most profound truths, the "secrets" of the universe, are contained in the most simple, basic facts of life. Breathing is one of these secrets. It is so fundamental, it seems so natural and effortless, we usually take it for granted. We don't realize its tremendous significance and potential power.

It is well known that you can go without food for weeks. You can survive without water for days. But a very few minutes without breath and you're dead. We all know this, so what's the point?

The point is that your entire future, your life itself, totally depends upon whether or not you receive your next inhalation. Nothing is more important to you than that next inhalation. Yet there is absolutely no guarantee that you're going to get it. Your guaranteed life expectancy is literally only one breath! All your wealth, all your possessions, all your relationships, power, prestige, hopes, and plans are useless unless you are breathing.

That is why the first principle in Kundalini Yoga is:

Value Your Breath

Each breath is given to you. "You" are not breathing; something is breathing in you. Think about it. From the moment you were born, up to this very moment in time, twenty-four hours every day, seven days a week, 365 days a year—-no holidays, no vacations, no time off; whether you are awake or asleep, conscious or unconscious, happy or unhappy; something breathes in you, keeping you alive.

Here comes a most significant thought: Some people call that amazing power, energy, or force that breathes in you: "GOD." Yes, it is true, the One Universal Intelligence that Generates, Organizes, and then Delivers or Destroys all creation is precisely what is breathing in each of us.

Hold on a minute, are we talking about religion here? No! Definitely not. Religion is how you choose (if you choose) to worship That-Which-Breathes-in-You.

Breath is the delicate thread that links you, the creature, to the One who created this entire universe (including you and me). Each inhalation you receive is a reminder, a reaffirmation of that divine presence in you.

"If there is anything Divine in you, it's your breath."
—Yogi Bhajan

In the Orient, it is said that when a child is born, the life-span is already predetermined, premeasured, preordained and predestined—not by years, but by the number of breaths allotted. Therefore, we can conclude, and rightfully so, if you breathe slower, you will live longer. You will also live healthier. A slower rate of breathing is much easier on the nervous system, the metabolism, and the digestion.

The rate and rhythm of the breath are intimately connected to our mental and emotional states. In fact, just as the emotions and the mind cause the breath to vary, by consciously controlling the breath we can gain control over the mind and the emotions. By slowing down the breath, we calm the mind and cool down our emotional energy.

The average rate of breathing for most people is about fifteen times per minute. When the rate of breathing increases, or if it becomes rapid and irregular, the mind also becomes disturbed and erratic. We already know this instinctively. In a movie, when we hear someone gasping, breathing heavily, even if we can't see them, we feel the tension, we assume they're upset. When we want to know if the baby is asleep, we listen for slow, even breathing.

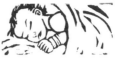

PRANA AND THE AIR

Yes, breath is life, but it isn't the air we breathe that keeps us alive. It is the subtle essence of the breath, carried to us by the air, that contains our life energy. This life energy is called prana. The prana that we receive with each breath is the same energy that was released when scientists split the atom. It is nothing new.

For thousands of years the yogis have worked with prana. Yogic breathing exercises are called pranayam. Prana is the basic building block of the universe. It is given to us with each inhalation. What could be more powerful?

When a person dies, the body still contains air. But the prana, the divine life force, has been withdrawn.

> ## Incoming breath of life
> ## is PRANA.
> ## Outgoing breath is called APANA.

More about apana later.

Principles to remember:

1. Your rate of breathing and your state of mind are inseparable.

2. The slower your rate of breathing, the more control you have over your mind.

Another principle to remember — especially later on when we talk about relaxation, is:

3. The mind follows the breath, and the body follows the mind.

PRANAYAM: CONSCIOUS BREATHING

My very first class with Yogi Bhajan consisted entirely of slow, long, deep breathing. He told me to lie down flat on my back on the floor (fortunately there was a mat) and start inhaling and exhaling as deeply as possible through my nose. Then he left the room! Forty-five minutes later he returned. That was my introduction to Kundalini Yoga.

21

Yogi Bhajan didn't give me any technical, detailed instructions. He just said to lie straight, keep my arms at my sides and breathe long and deep through the nose — consciously. Conscious breathing means focusing your attention on each inhalation and exhalation. It's a very different experience from simply letting the breath "happen" as we do most of the time.

The most fundamental yogic breathing technique is simply Long Deep Breathing.

LONG DEEP BREATHING

What is the effect of Long Deep Breathing? It will calm the mind, balance the emotions, and harmonize body, mind, and spirit. It is used in meditation, and in the practice of yoga exercises. Long Deep Breathing can be used in every-day situations where you want to be in control of your emotions, able to think clearly and act effectively. Remember, the slower you breathe, the calmer your mind. Used in conjunction with positive affirmation, Long Deep Breathing becomes a very dynamic self-healing tool.

So, let's do it! Sit up straight, or you can even lie down flat on your back. Close your eyes. Tune in with **ONG NAMO GURU DEV NAMO**. *(See Tuning In.)* The main requirement is that the spine must not be bent anywhere; it must be straight. We're going to use Long Deep Breathing as the pranayam with a Meditation for Universal Wisdom. *(See facing page.)*

You can use Long Deep Breathing as a guided meditation for many aspects of self-healing. Choose your own list of qualities to meditate on and consciously receive and accept whatever concept you choose with each inhalation. Then release, or let go of the opposite quality with each exhalation For example:

INHALE	EXHALE
health	disease
strength	weakness
energy	fatigue
faith	fear
peace	tension

MEDITATION FOR UNIVERSAL WISDOM

To focus your energy on the quality of wisdom, with your hands resting on your knees (palms can be up or down), curl your forefingers and capture the tip of the nail of the forefingers with the pad of the first joint of your thumbs. The other three fingers of each hand are straight and close together. Your arms are straight, with no bend in the elbows, but they are not rigid. Your body is like a pyramid, balanced, symmetrical, and stable. The majestic yogi!

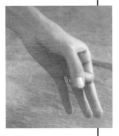

Inhale deeply through your nose. Feel as though you are pulling the breath down into your navel center. As the breath then starts to fill the lungs, your diaphragm will expand. You can think of the abdominal area as a balloon. Keep inhaling until your lungs have taken in all they can hold. Your chest will be expanded.

Keep track of the breath and feel it as it comes in and goes out. Breathe deeply, feel the breath going all the way down to the navel point. When you exhale, empty the lungs completely.

Use your total lung capacity, make every inhale and every exhale as long and full and complete as you can. It will soon take greater concentration to maintain the depth of the breath — because as the breath slows down, the mind slows down also, and tends to put you to sleep. (This principle comes in handy when you want to go to sleep at night. We'll talk more about this in the chapter on Sleep.) Try to stay alert and continue to make each breath full and deep.

Keep your abdominal muscles relaxed during long deep breathing. The abdomen will move naturally with the breath. It's the diaphragm that's doing all the work. Consciously feel yourself taking in and absorbing universal wisdom with each inhalation, and getting rid of doubt and confusion with each exhalation.

Continue for three minutes. See how peaceful and mentally clear you feel after only three minutes! Of course, you can do long deep breathing for longer periods of time (eleven minutes, thirty-one minutes, or more), but as usual, we recommend moderation. Begin with short sessions and gradually increase your time.

It seems so simple, but believe me, it works! You already have that infinite creative flow of eternal power within you. This is one way to use it. Keep remembering that breath is life, and therefore breath can rejuvenate and regenerate.

CORPSE POSE

You can do Long Deep Breathing (or any pranayam) lying flat on your back, keeping your body in a straight line, arms down at your sides, palms facing up. Then you can tell your friends you mastered one of the Hatha Yoga Asanas (postures)! It is called Corpse Pose. This position gives optimum support to the spine (which has all 72,000 nerves attached to the twenty-six main vertebrae) and allows the free-flowing of energy throughout the body.

LINKING THE BREATH WITH MANTRA

One of the simplest but nevertheless most powerful ways to meditate on the breath is to think the sound "SAT" with every inhalation and think the sound "NAM" with every exhalation. Hear the syllables in your mind. (Suuuuuuuuut... rhymes with "but," Naaaaaaaaam, rhymes with "calm.") Mentally create these sounds. Take your time. Take ten long, deep, full breaths, meditating on each breath with the infinite sound of SAT NAM.

Why do we use those particular syllables? SAT NAM instantly attunes us to our highest Self. SAT NAM affirms that "Truth is our Identity." It translates as: "Truth is God's Name." We'll talk much more about mantra later, meanwhile, a little explanation about a big concept:

"In the beginning was the Word, and the Word was with God, and the Word was God."[1]
SAT NAM

SAT NAM is a Bij Mantra, or "seed sound." SAT means Truth, the ultimate, unchanging, Universal Truth. NAM means name, or identity. When we say "SAT NAM" to each other, we are acknowledging our mutual divine identity. And, at least for that brief moment, we are united, "one in the spirit." There are no barriers, no walls of fear or separation between us. By using Sat Nam as a greeting

(I even have it on my voice mail) we have attuned ourselves to our highest consciousness, at least for a moment. After that we can decide to disagree about anything we want! But at least we have established a basis of communication that is in total harmony and acceptance. I think it's called love.

EXPAND YOUR LUNG CAPACITY

SAT NAM

When your mind is calm, meditative, and under your control, your rate of breathing will be slow, steady and calm. So, it is logical that by breathing slowly and steadily you will calm your mind. Yes, to repeat, it's a fact: As you change your rate of breathing, you change your state of mind. To breathe more slowly, it is necessary to have a larger lung capacity. One of the first things we work on is increasing the lung capacity. The fastest way to achieve that is by practicing Breath of Fire.

BREATH OF FIRE

Here is a pranayam that will not only increase your lung capacity (so you can easily breathe slower and deeper) but it will also:

- Strengthen your nervous system
- Purify your bloodstream
- Energize, stimulate, and wake you up!
- Increase your vitality

This pranayam is called Breath of Fire. It is one of the first things I teach my beginning students. I want to teach it to you right now. So please "Tune In" with **ONG NAMO GURU DEV NAMO**, and we'll be ready to begin.

Let us sit properly like yogis, in Sukhasan, easy cross-legged pose. If you become too uncomfortable, try sitting on your heels (Vajra Asan — Rock Pose), or sit in a chair, or lie on the floor. The main thing is you are going to BREATHE CONSCIOUSLY, with your spine straight.

Interlace your fingers in your lap. Ideally, apply "Venus Lock." Venus Lock will help you contain the increased energy from the additional prana that you are going to bring into your body when you do Breath of Fire.

Look at the illustration carefully. Note that the thumbs are not crossed. The hand position is opposite for males and females. *(Female lock illustrated.)* The tip of one thumb is pressing firmly into the web between the thumb and forefinger of the other hand, while the opposite thumb is pressing the fleshy mound between the thumb and the wrist. Make sure to alternate the fingers. You don't want to have two fingers from the same hand next to each other.

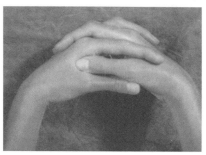

Venus Lock

HOW TO DO BREATH OF FIRE

Breath of Fire is simply a rapid and powerful breath through the nose. To learn it, be sure your spine is straight, keep your mouth closed, and breathe rapidly through the nose. Inhalation and exhalation will be about equal. (It is *not* the Hatha Yoga breath "Bastrika" which emphasizes the exhalation and focuses on the lower stomach muscles.)

Inhale and lift your chest and hold it still. Exhale and pull in on your navel. Note that the upper abdominals and the diaphragm move as the navel point pulls in. The breath is powered from the navel to the diaphragm. In the beginning, you may find it helpful to think primarily about the exhalation which is synchronized with the pulling in of the navel.

Listen to the sound of your breath. Imagine that you are making the sound track for a film showing twenty-seven steam engines going uphill.

Start out slowly as you're learning, until you get used to the rhythm and can easily coordinate the breath with the movement of your navel point. Then pick up speed until you're breathing approximately 120 to 180 times per minute.

Listen to the sound of your breath. Imagine that you are making the sound track for a film showing twenty-seven steam engines going uphill.

On each exhalation, pull your navel point in toward the back of your spine. On each inhalation, release it. Don't pause in between. When Breath of Fire is done correctly, it is an easy breath. The muscles dance in rhythm and you stay energized rather than becoming tired.

Breath of Fire is not hyperventilation. In hyperventilation, the breathing is deep and erratic. The upper chest is not held supended, and usually people are "chest breathing" or they may be reverse breathing, in other words exhaling with the navel pushed out instead of pulled in.

Continue Breath of Fire, breathing rapidly and continuously in and out without pausing, for about thirty seconds for your first practice session. Keep your shoulders relaxed, keep your face relaxed. Allow yourself to do Breath of Fire without tension. Keep your spine straight, but not rigid.

Do not inhale or exhale through your mouth to catch your breath. If you should start to feel you are running out of breath and you think you must stop, simply take a few long, slow, deep breaths through your nose until you feel ready to resume. Then try again.

Don't pause or hold your breath on either the inhalation or exhalation. Breath of Fire is one continuous breath. Even though it may seem like a lot of inhalations and exhalations, it is considered to be all one breath, from the time you start, to the time you stop. That is why it is so marvelously effective in calming your mind. (The slower the breath, the calmer the mind.) When you do Breath of Fire for even just one minute, the

---

If I were writing a commercial for Breath of Fire, I'd say:

Are your nerves "frayed"? Do you fly off the handle at the slightest provocation?

TRY THIS WEEK'S SPECIAL PRANAYAM: "BREATH OF FIRE"

- Breath of Fire virtually insulates your nerves. It coats them with an invisible but powerful protective pranic cushion that can last for days.
- Practiced regularly, Breath of Fire is guaranteed by the Yogis to end any embarrassing temper tantrum habit.
- Amaze your friends and family with your calm, serene disposition.

Well, you get the idea. Breath of Fire does wonders for strengthening your 72,000 nerves and because it expands your lung capacity, enabling you to breathe slowly, it activates your intuition.

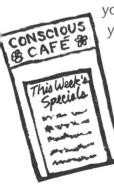

effect is as if you had taken only one breath during that whole minute! Breathing less than four times per minute puts you into a meditative state. Furthermore, breathing slowly increases the flow of your inner intuitive guidance.

BREATH AND INTUITION

Here's how it works: When you breathe less than eight times per minute, you stimulate the secretion of your pituitary gland. Not only is the pituitary the master gland of the body, but it is also the gateway, the control panel for your intuition. The more your pituitary secretes, the more active and accessible your intuition becomes. This means that you become more aware of actions you need to take. You will find your inner guidance, that direct, instantaneous awareness of "simply knowing," becoming more frequent, stronger, and clearer. Through Kundalini Yoga meditations you will also learn how to use your meditative mind and how to call upon your intuition at will.

PHYSICAL EFFECTS

Breath of Fire is a cleansing and purifying breath, so if you are doing Breath of Fire for the first time, you may notice some physical effects. Especially if your bloodstream is holding a lot of toxins, you may feel slightly giddy or dizzy in the process. Don't worry about it, just keep on breathing. It may be uncomfortable but it is not harmful. You are simply feeling the poisons coming to the surface where they can be eliminated.

In any cleansing process (such as a very strict cleansing diet or fast) you may feel weak at first, possibly even a little worse than before you started. By continuing, you will get rid of those toxins that would otherwise stay locked up inside your body until some fine day they decide to reveal themselves, when you "get sick."

Other symptoms can occur when you start doing Breath of Fire. You may feel heat or cold inside your nostrils. You may feel a pressure at the root of the nose. Some people feel "itchy" or tingly. Some people feel none of the above. The various sensations are incidental, temporary adjustments made by your body. Ignore them. Breath of Fire generates a lot of heat so it warms up the body. (Try it on a cold day!) Since it usually increases your circulation, women should not practice Breath of Fire during their monthly period.

You can make Breath of Fire even more powerful by adding the mantra (mentally hearing the sounds), *Wahe Guru, Wahe Guru, Wahe Guru...(pronounced Waa Hay G'roo—see Pronunciatian Guide)* repeated rapidly over and over in rhythm with your breath. **Wahe Guru** means "Wow, God is Great!" It is a mantra of ecstasy. Or you can silently repeat the Bij Mantra, **SAT NAM**, six times, "*Sat Nam, Sat Nam, Sat Nam, Sat Nam, Sat Nam, Sat Nam*, then add: *Wahe Guru!* to each cycle.

SAT NAM
SAT NAM
SAT NAM
SAT NAM
SAT NAM
SAT NAM
WAHE GURU

HOMEWORK ASSIGNMENT

Be kind to yourself. Start practicing Breath of Fire on a regular basis. Every single day, sit down with a watch or a timer, and simply do it. Give yourself five minutes every day, starting with 30-second segments. Take a few long, deep breaths in-between when you need to. Keep practicing! Work your way up to longer segments each day and by the end of a week you will be able to do Breath of Fire comfortably for two minutes without stopping. Of course, practice on an empty stomach! You don't want to eat anything within one hour before any session, and eat only very lightly within two hours prior to doing Kundalini Yoga.

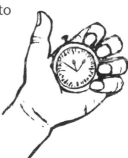

Breath of Fire is a very important factor in many Kundalini Yoga exercises, so PRACTICE, PRACTICE, PRACTICE! Discover how energizing it is, and how good it makes you feel!

TWO NOSTRILS ARE BETTER THAN ONE !

We've talked about the breath and its relationship to our state of mind. We've learned the two most fundamental pranayams: Breath of Fire, the pranayam that strengthens the nervous system and expands your lung capacity, and Long Deep Breathing.

Now let's talk about why you have two nostrils and then learn how to use them individually.

Your body temperature is regulated by the flow of the prana through alternate nostrils. They function somewhat like an air-conditioning unit and a furnace, turning on and off, switching back and forth from heating to cooling every two and a half hours, keeping your temperature normal and your energies in balance.

Your pituitary gland — the master gland of the body — serves as the thermostat to control the switches. The left nostril draws in the cooling, soothing, mind-expanding energy of the moon. It is the "water" element. The right nostril draws on the sun's energy. This is for vitality, activity, and mental alertness; it heats the body. You can experiment right now and find out which of your nostrils is working. Place a finger underneath your nose and gently exhale. You will discover that the air is flowing mostly out of only one nostril.

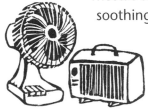

The right nostril controls our energy level and the left controls our emotions. Consequently, if we are tired, breathing long and deep through the right nostril will give us added energy. Breathing through the left nostril can calm us down when we are upset and emotional, angry, frightened, or just generally disturbed.

Although your body has its own rhythm for automatically alternating nostrils for breathing, there are times when you will benefit from consciously controlling this function. Many pranayams use one, both, or alternate nostrils, depending upon the effect desired.

LEFT NOSTRIL BREATHING: CALM DOWN AND COOL OFF

If you're upset, angry, agitated, mentally/emotionally disturbed, or just plain moving too fast and feeling pressured and stressed out, try this:

Find a private place where no one will disturb you, and take five minutes for this pranayam.

Sit with your spine straight. Using the thumb of the right hand, keeping the other fingers together and pointing straight upward like antennae, close your right nostril. Begin long deep breathing in and out through the left nostril only.

TWENTY-SIX long deep breaths through the left nostril will do the job. When you are calm, then you can decide how to deal with whatever situation requires your action, because you won't be triggered into any emotional knee-jerk response.

ALTERNATE NOSTRIL BREATHING:
ENERGIZE AND CALM THE NERVOUS SYSTEM

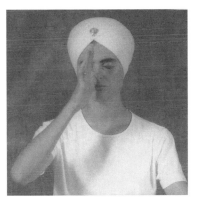

Here's a breathing technique using alternate nostrils to soothe and calm and at the same time energize your whole nervous system. It works because the energy of your nervous system is directly proportional to your breath.

In only three to five minutes you can revitalize your whole nervous system. This particular technique can come in handy when you feel "off-center" and yet have to function at your job, or in school, or at home. Suppose you have an important business meeting scheduled but you're feeling extremely nervous and irritable. This pranayam can help you calm down so you can be effective in your communication at that meeting. Here's how:

Sit comfortably with your spine straight. Use your thumb and index finger of the right hand. Make a "U" of your thumb and forefinger. Use the thumb to close off the right nostril while breathing in or out through the left nostril, and the index finger to close off the left nostril while breathing in or out through the right nostril. Keep your other hand in your lap, or resting on your left knee.

The breath sequence goes like this:

Close the left nostril; inhale deeply through the right nostril. At the completion of inhalation, close the right nostril and exhale through the left one. Now inhale through the left nostril fully and deeply. Then close the left nostril and exhale through the right one. Again, inhale through the right nostril and exhale through the left. Continue this breathing pattern for three to five minutes.

Breathe fully on both inhalation and exhalation cycles. After three to five minutes, inhale deeply, hold the breath in for a few seconds, then lower the hand and exhale through both nostrils. Relax and feel great!

"THE ONE MINUTE YOGI"

Catch yourself breathing!

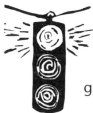

When you're walking down the street, sitting in a restaurant, opening your mail, waiting for the light to change, during the TV commercial— catch yourself breathing! Wake up to the fact that you are breathing and therefore you are alive. Remember WHO is giving you each inhalation, and say "Thank You!"

Meditation on the breath is one of the
highest forms of meditation.
Never Underestimate The Power of Your Breath.

PRANA

God is not off somewhere
Inaccessible and far.
Each inhalation confirms God's presence in you
Right here, right now, right where you are.

Why should Truth between man and God
Not be spoken aloud?
What is that lie man told to man
To keep him from feeling proud?-

Proud of the God
Who breathes within —
Divine Being of Light
Covered with skin.

When a body "dies" there's still air inside
What's gone is PRANA, essence of life itself,
Can't be bought with the greatest wealth.

Prana, subtle essence of God
Primal energy released when the atom was split
Basic building block of the universe
All human life depends on it.

God's loving gift of life constantly renewed,
Power to hear and see and say—
How you choose to use it liberates or condemns you
Moment to moment, every day.

Take away Prana,   Breathe slowly, breathe deeply
Only a shell remains   Your mind will be calm
No matter what wealth   Besides, you'll live longer
Or material gains.   And seldom be wrong.

Value your breath, it's sacred, it's pure
If there's anything Divine in you — it's your breath for sure!

5

Mantra

"Magic Words"

HISTORY, MYTH, LEGEND

One story I read when I was a child told about a beautiful princess who was held prisoner in a tower. She gained her freedom by guessing the name of her captor. (It was "Rumplestilskin," in case you've forgotten.) Ali Baba and the Forty Thieves found the treasure cave by saying the magic words, "Open sesame," whereupon a hidden door miraculously appeared. These words were, in effect mantras. It's no fairy tale, it's a fact, when you know the "magic" words, you can find the hidden treasure!

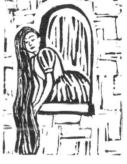

The scientific use of sound to affect consciousness is called Mantra Yoga. Next to breathing (necessary for any endeavor), the use of Mantra is the most important aspect of the practice of Kundalini Yoga.

"MAN" means mind. "TRA" means to tune the vibration (just as one tunes the strings of a guitar). Mantra is a sound current which tunes and controls mental vibration. It is the "directive psyche," a word or words, combinations of syllables, which help focus the mind. Such words have enormous power.

"What does it mean to master a mantra? When you have repeated it so much, so often, and so well that you hear it within your being, and it comes handy to you — especially at the moment of death — you have mastered a mantra."[1]

"Mantram siddhyam, siddhyam Parameshwaram." He who masters mantra, masters God Himself.

Claims for mantras may seem like miracles, but mantras are actually formulas that work according to physical and metaphysical laws.

"Repeating a mantra (aloud) restructures the patterns in the mind that allow experience. Silence makes you aware of the many experiences in the mind."[2]

GOOD VIBES !

We live in a sea of energy. Energy vibrates. Everything in the manifest creation is vibrating. Even seemingly solid, inanimate objects are constantly vibrating. They are simply vibrating at a slower or lower frequency than animate objects. Some vibrations are audible, they are sounds we can hear with our ears. Thoughts are silent sounds, electromagnetic vibrations. The higher the frequency, the less dense and more etheric the quality of the vibrations we hear and speak, the more our own vibrational frequency is raised. Raising our own vibration brings us closer to experiencing and merging with the highest vibration of all, GOD, the original cause of the creativity of the universe.

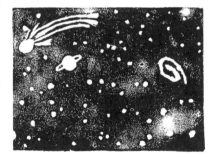

Our entire universe was built on sound, on vibration. Putting it poetically: God spoke, and the world came into being. Or, more precisely, God vibrated, and all the universes and worlds, solar systems, oceans, land, and sky, and the myriad of beings that inhabit them appeared.

There's a vibratory frequency that corresponds to everything in the universe. By vibrating a particular combination of sounds, you

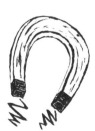

tune in to various levels of intelligence, or consciousness. Situations, people, and events respond to the signals you send out. The vibratory frequency of a mantra draws to you whatever you are vibrating. You are like a magnet attracting vibrations to you by what you send out.

Chanting mantras, either silently or aloud, is a conscious method of controlling and directing your mind. Happiness or sorrow, joy or regret are vibratory frequencies in the mind. We can call them attitudes, or beliefs, but fundamentally, they are vibratory frequencies or thought waves. They determine the kind of program our mind "plays." Which scenario we choose to hold on to becomes our vibration, defines how we feel and what we project to others. We can exercise our right to choose at any time.

When we chant a mantra we are choosing to invoke the positive power contained in those particular syllables. Whether it's for prosperity, peace of mind, increasing intuition, or any of the other multitude of possible benefits inherent in mantras, simply by chanting them we are setting vibrations into motion that shall have an effect. It doesn't actually matter if we understand the meaning of the sounds or not.

We are creating with every word we speak, and even with every word we think. Words are like boomerangs, every vibration we send out shall come back to us sooner or later. We get what we tune in to.

YOUR PERSONAL MANTRA

Some people think they need a personal mantra. Actually whatever mantra you chant becomes your personal mantra! As the Master of Kundalini Yoga himself has said:

"The word 'mantra' means mental vibration to the infinite mind. It's a direct connection between God and you. Mantra is personal. It affects us personally. Its vibrations are personal. Because, if it is your heartline telephone, and you're dialing it, and you're reaching God, it's not mine, and it's not anybody else's. It's yours."[3]

"The conversation of the mind with the soul is the essence of mantra. Mantra means to project and protect the mind. It gives the mind direction... When language and rhythm blend to instill a thought at the deepest level, it is a powerful mantra. It is sacred speech. It is a special use of language."[4]

"Day by day in every way, I'm getting better and better."

THE POWER OF POSITIVE THINKING WORKS

Dr. Emil Coue created a major sensation in the early part of the twentieth century when his affirmation, "Day by day in every way, I'm getting better and better," became the rage. The concept of positive thinking seemed revolutionary! Dr Normal Vincent Peale reached millions of people with his famous best seller, *The Power of Positive Thinking*. Dale Carnegie applied these same principles in his *How to Win Friends and Influence People*. These men discovered and taught the creative power of words. The yogis understood this power very well.

In yogic terms, positive thinking is the substitution of a positive thought wave in the mind for a negative one. Positive affirmation is a form of mantra. Positive words can heal, uplift, and inspire. The other side of the coin is that careless, unkind, negative words can hurt. Words are like sharp tools, which

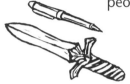

people can use like a surgeon's scalpel to save a life, or a butcher knife to kill.

It's been said, "The pen is mightier than the sword."[5] Each word we think or say literally starts a creative process in the universe. Don't underestimate your power of the Word. Be careful what you say. In fact, be especially careful what you pray for, you're liable to get it!

WHY DON'T WE CHANT IN ENGLISH?

Sometimes we do. However, to achieve the greatest impact on our consciousness, we use mantras in Gurbani, a language based on the science of NAAD. These mantras are the most effective. Affirmations and mantras in English certainly have an effect on our minds and emotions, but the most profound changes in our consciousness take place on a much deeper level. The actual chemistry of the brain has to change for us to experience Infinity.

THE SCIENCE OF NAAD

"Naad means harmony, a process of harmony through which the "Aad," the Infinity, can be experienced. Naad is the basic sound for all languages through all times. This sound comes from one common source called the sound current. It is the universal code behind language and therefore behind human communication.

"The Science of Naad works between the movement of the tongue in the mouth, through language, and chemicals in the brain. There is no nerve connecting system from one section of the brain to another. There is no wiring, instead there is a solution, neuro-transmission fluid. Different chemical liquids are secreted from all different parts of the brain. Messages are transmitted very fast from each part of the brain through the fluids which are called "Naad Namodam Rasaa." Naad means communication, namodam means addressing and rasaa means juice..." [6]

COMBINATION LOCK

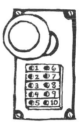

In addition to the vibrations set in motion, something else happens when you chant. This is really important. There are eighty-four meridian points, or pressure points in the roof of the mouth. Every time you speak you stimulate them with the tongue. By stimulating these pressure points on the upper palate in a particular sequence, using the right access code, you increase the secretion of the hypothalamus gland and actually bring about a change in the permutation and combination of your brain cells. You affect the chemistry of the brain. When giving instructions for chanting certain mantras, Yogi Bhajan has been specific in saying,"Use the tip of your tongue."

"You can feel the upper palate with the tongue and experience its different surfaces. There are two rows of meridian points on the upper palate and on the gum behind the upper teeth. The tongue stimulates those meridian points, and they in turn stimulate the hypothalamus which makes the pineal gland radiate. When the pineal gland radiates, it creates an impulsation in the pituitary gland. When the pituitary gland gives impulsation, the entire glandular system secretes and a human being obtains bliss. This is the science."[7]

It's as if you have an electronic, computerized security system in your mouth. Punch in the right code on the upper palate and you gain entry to the brain and your inner chambers of higher consciousness!

When we chant, we are also using prana, the life force of the universe ("atomic energy") to create a sound current. No wonder chanting is so powerful.

TECHNICAL TERMS
(in case you're interested)

KINDS OF SOUND

We usually think of sound as audible but sound can also be subtle. It can be vibrated with one part of you, or with your whole self.
The yogis define several distinct kinds of sound or shabd.

• **BHAKREE:** Using the tip of the tongue to form the syllables aloud is called "Bhakree." It is the easiest way to chant.

• **KHANT:** This is the sound current that you hear in your mind when you read silently, without moving your lips. It is subliminal vocalization. The "sound" is silent, but the syllables vibrate at your Throat Chakra (Fifth Center of Consciousness).

• **HARDAY:** This is the sound current that vibrates in the heart. This is how a mother can "hear" the voice of her wounded son crying out from the battlefield six thousand miles away.

• **ANAHAT:** This sound current is sometimes called the "Unstruck Melody." It is when the mantra resounds in every atom and fiber of your being; every nerve is attuned to it. Its vibration becomes a part of you. It is an inner sound. It is created when the sound is produced from the navel center (Nabhee) using the tip of the tongue. This combination triggers the higher glands to produce the "nectar of bliss," amrit.

Because of its power, the science of mantra was kept a carefully guarded secret in the Orient for thousands of years, but Yogi Bhajan has openly taught the "secret code" words and the techology to open the doors of our inner perception. His attitude is, "What is that Truth between God and man which cannot be spoken aloud?"

In the *Things To Do* section you will find the mantras I've selected to share with you, with detailed instructions on how to chant them for the best results.

6
Conquer Your Mind,
You Conquer the World[1]

"Mind your own business"
"Mind your manners"
"Mind over matter"
"Never mind..."
"Mind your mother!"
"I don't mind if I do..."

*C*ontrary to popular belief, your mind is not you. Your identity is much more permanent than that. Think how often your mind changes (or you "change your mind"). But your identity doesn't change. You're still "you," no matter what your mind is thinking, planning, advising, or arguing about.

Just as your physical body is not "you," neither is your mind. It is equally a vehicle, to help you function here on earth. It's supposed to be your useful servant, your friend, not your boss!

Have you ever watched your mind? It can be a very educational experience! The very fact that "you" can watch your mind demonstrates that the mind is not you. The mind is something separate from you, an "object" that you can observe.

Mastering the mind is one of the aims of Kundalini Yoga (or any yoga) because until you can control the mind, you can't get beyond it to liberation. Liberation is the experience of your own infinity, and lies beyond the mind.

That doesn't mean that you throw away the mind, or destroy it, or suppress it. In fact, you want to make the mind sharper, clearer, and even more useful than ever.

You can use the breath to control the mind, for *the mind always follows the breath* and the body follows the mind. Self-mastery starts with the breath. If you haven't already done so, please go back and read the chapter on breath. And look up the *Basic Breath Series* that is especially recommended to help make the mind sharp and clear.

> **"The mind becomes a monster when it becomes your master. The mind is an angel when it is your servant."**
>
> —Yogi Bhajan

THREE MINDS ARE BETTER THAN ONE

CONSCIOUS MINDS

You actually have three minds (no wonder sometimes it's so hard to "make up your mind"). Count 'em:

1. The first mind is your protector, It acts as an alarm system. It is called the Negative Mind. It warns you of the danger or disadvantage in any upcoming situation or decision. It's valuable. You need it. It's the mind that keeps you from stepping in front of moving trains. But you don't want to make it the final authority in your life. When carried to extremes it could make you afraid of trains that are standing still.

2. The second mind is the Positive Mind. This is the mind that reveals to you the possible gain or advantage you can get out of a situation. It should start communicating with you within a few seconds, almost immediately after the Negative Mind has given its input. By all means listen to your Positive Mind, but don't act yet. After you receive all the pros and cons, you still don't know enough to make a decision, until you find out what your third mind has to say.

3. Your third mind is your Neutral Mind. It is not clouded by fear and insecurity. It's not fooled by wishful thinking. Its only bias is to provide the best, most conscious, wise solution to any problem. This is the mind you can trust. It has your best interests at heart (and in mind).

Whether it's in your business or personal relationships, health, or where to spend your vacation, in order to determine what's really best for you now and for the future, you not only need to be aware of what opinion is held by the Positive Mind and what opinion is held by the Negative Mind, you also need to consult your Neutral or Meditative Mind for a decision.

The practice of Kundalini Yoga helps to develop the Neutral or Meditative Mind so that it becomes more and more powerful and active and you can go to it very quickly for problem-solving advice .

SUB-CONSCIOUS MIND

In addition to your conscious mind, you also have a very active sub-conscious mind and deeper than that, a vast subterranean area of the unconscious.

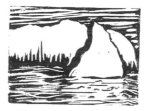

The conscious mind is just the tip of the iceberg. Most of what motivates us is below the surface. A huge proportion of our behavior is dictated by promptings we get from the sub-conscious mind, which doesn't know fact from fiction. It is a catch-all for the verbal input and even the nonverbal input we receive constantly. It doesn't judge what it receives, and pretty much accepts everything as gospel, coloring our habits of thinking, speaking, and acting - with its limited understanding.

You can use the gullibility of the subconscious to heal yourself. If you repeat "I am perfectly healthy" over and over, even while you're running a fever of 103°,

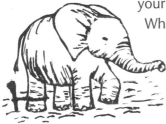

your subconscious will believe it and you will heal faster. Whatever the subconscious mind believes, the body tends to manifest. "As above, so below." Another reason why positive affirmation works! But until we get rid of the fear and the neuroses in the subconscious we are very handicapped in our lives.

Think about an elephant. They say elephants never forget (neither do people). Have you ever wondered why a huge two thousand pound elephant will stand so obediently in one place, tied to a short stake in the ground, held only by a thin chain around its ankle? The elephant doesn't try to move, because he has been programmed to believe he can't.

How? Simple. The baby elephant is tied to the stake when he is very young. Whenever he tries to move, the chain bites into his leg. He can't get away, because he's not strong enough. Every time he tries to move, he gets hurt — a lot. The elephant very quickly catches on to the fact that moving is painful. In order to avoid getting hurt, he gives up trying. Even after he has grown to full size, and could easily tear out the chain, along with the post, and probably the whole circus tent, this gigantic, powerful elephant doesn't even try to get free, because he believes he can't.

Similarly, we let ourselves suffer from low self-esteem, think of ourselves as "sinners," and accept defeat or failure because our subconscious minds have accepted these false concepts. We believe things that we've been told, things we may not even consciously remember hearing.

You can go to a psychiatrist or psychologist and spend a lot of hours and a lot of dollars to sort through and examine the self-defeating attitudes in the subconscious. Or you can use the techniques of meditation and mantra, dissolve the pain, and just get rid of the garbage that is clogging up your subconscious mind.

WHERE DO THOUGHTS COME FROM?

The intellect releases one thousand thoughts per wink of the eye. Yes, everyone—genius, idiot, and the rest of us in between, each person gets one thousand thoughts every time he or she blinks! And these thoughts have to be processed.

WHERE DO THOUGHTS GO?

Each thought becomes either a
        • Feeling   • Emotion or   • Desire

When your desires don't work out, you feel upset. When you don't have intuition to guide you, mostly you won't get your desires fulfilled. Unfulfilled desire becomes neurosis, and that can develop into psychosis.

All thoughts and feelings go into the subconscious. When that gets filled up to overflowing, the excess spills into the unconscious, and that becomes the source of nightmares for you. Once they fall into the unconscious, those attitudes, feelings, and habits are extremely difficult to reach to change or modify, much less eliminate. That is why it is so essential for sanity and survival to clear out the subconscious on a regular basis, to prevent that "overload" of thoughts and feelings going into the unconscious.

DEEP CLEANING IS NOT JUST FOR SPRING

Sadhana, the daily practice of meditation/mantra, is one of the best, most efficient housecleaning services for the subconscious corridors of your mind. Because sadhana is a cleansing process, you have to be prepared for the dust to fly. That's why meditating is not necessarily blissful. Old fears, buried anger, deep negative emotions are brought up to the surface by the process so that the power of the mantra can dissolve them. (One vibration dissolving/absorbing the other.) Otherwise they remain buried and become more deeply entrenched in your subconscious, or become a permanent part of your unconscious, causing you even greater suffering and unhappiness.

FOCUS ON MANTRA

When painful, negative thoughts and feelings come out, let them go on by. Keep bringing your mind back to focus on the mantra you are chanting. And keep on chanting! This is substituting the positive thought wave of the mantra for the negative thought waves in your mind. The high vibration of mantra, like a good detergent, dissolves the greasy, grimy, painful thought waves. It's a process. Go through it.

Supposing you're just sitting and worrying, or you wake up with doubt or fear in your mind. "You can, by your free will, create the thought that 'God is with me. God and me, me and God are One.' To every thought that comes, if you meet it with this thought, you will be plus, not minus....Because you and God together will be meeting the thought, and you will win."[2]

HOW TO WIN

Choose an affirmation or mantra *(See Chapter on Mantra and also the Persian Wheel Mantra)* to use whenever you catch your mind in a negative mode. Use it so much that it becomes "second nature" to you. Let that sound current carry away your worry or confusion, doubt or fear!

Here are two simple sample sound currents
to clear your mind:

"GOD AND ME, ME AND GOD ARE ONE"

Be sure to affirm this with conscious acceptance that it's true!

"ANG SANG WAHE GURU"

(pronounced *Ung Sung Waahay G'roo*)

("God is in every limb, every part, every fiber of my being.")

7
Mysterious Kundalini

"Where there's mastery,
there's no mystery."

—Yogi Bhajan

Kundalini energy is real. It is powerful, and it's flowing through your body right now. It feeds your entire nervous system. For centuries, knowledge about it was kept secret because of its tremendous power. Because of the secrecy and lack of accurate information, many false representations have been put forth by otherwise respectable, so-called authorities. Sometimes people have had spontaneous experiences of the kundalini energy rising, but have not had the preparation and understanding to properly integrate and use the energy. That is why Yogi Bhajan's teachings are so valuable and important. Under his guidance as master of Kundalini Yoga, working with the kundalini energy becomes simple, the raising of the kundalini happens very easily, and the positive integration of the talents inherent in the various chakras takes place almost automatically. Using his method of teaching, practically anyone can practice Kundalini Yoga. (If I can do it, anybody can.)

Let me repeat, raising the kundalini is relatively simple. Keeping it flowing so that all the energy centers (chakras) are open and balanced is more of a challenge. To understand the value of this, we need to know more about the chakras and especially the function of the pineal and pituitary glands. *(See chapter on Chakras.)* So, bear with me through this next "scientific" section. Learn how the glands, the chakras, and the "mysterious" kundalini all work together to impact your awareness. And you can learn some yogic terms.

First of all, the word kundalini (feminine gender) literally means, "the curl of the lock of hair of the beloved." It is a metaphor, a poetic way of describing the flow of energy and consciousness which already exists within each one of us. Since ancient times, sacred truths have been hidden from the common man by using symbols and metaphors to pass along the knowledge.

Have you ever noticed the symbol printed on the prescription you get from your doctor? It's call a "Caduceus." It represents the flow of kundalini energy. This ancient symbol of the medical profession shows two serpents intertwined around a staff. But, kundalini is not snakes! It's just that in mythology and folklore, serpents are often associated with wisdom, and the route the kundalini energy travels as it goes up and down the spine is serpentine. The Caduceus represents the rising of the kundalini energy through two nerve channels that intertwine around the central nerve of the spinal column. These two nerves act as main conductors. One of them is called the Ida, the other, the Pingala. Each of them makes two and one-half turns around the central column of the spine (Shushmana), as they spiral upwards from the base of the spine. The kundalini energy they carry feeds the entire nervous system. The Ida and the Pingala conduct the basic positive and negative, solar and lunar energies of the body.

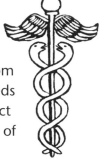

The Ida, the nerve which ends at the left nostril, brings in the cooling, soothing, mind-expanding energy of the moon. The Pingala, ending in the right nostril, brings in the stimulating, energizing, heating energy of the sun. In addition to the kundalini energy which is already flowing in us, there is a vast reservoir of untapped, or "dormant" kundalini stored under the fourth vertebra of the spinal column.

Through the practice of Kundalini Yoga, we stimulate and release this unused kundalini energy, and allow it (it is never forced) to rise up the central column of the spine until it reaches the top of the skull, activating the secretion of the pineal gland. This brings about a major change of consciousness. When this energy returns down the Ida and Pingala and activates and balances the various energy centers, there is a major change in the person's life. Although there are cases of the kundalini rising spontaneously, without purposeful spiritual practice, your reservoir of kundalini energy usually remains dormant throughout your entire life. It's like having a racing car and never getting out of first gear!

RAISING YOUR KUNDALINI

Raising your kundalini is not difficult. It happens so naturally when you practice Kundalini Yoga that you may not even recognize the actual moment that it happens. If you're expecting bells to ring, cannons to go off or lights to flash, forget it. Seeing visions, hearing sounds, having some physical sensation might sometimes happen,

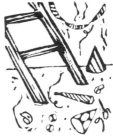

and could seem quite impressive, but it can also be very misleading. Such phenomena are not the goal of the practice of Kundalini Yoga. There may be no physical sign at all, or possibly just a very slight indication. In case you do experience such things, don't let yourself get sidetracked. They don't prove anything. They are not the criteria for whether the kundalini has risen. Yogi Bhajan calls them "glitter at the bottom of the ladder."[1]

Swami Vivekananda said,

"Wherever there was any manifestation of what is ordinarily called supernatural power or wisdom, there a little current of kundalini must have found its way into the shushmana. Only, in the vast majority of such cases, people had ignorantly stumbled on some practice which set free a minute portion of the coiled up kundalini. All worship, consciously or unconsciously, leads to this end."[2]

49

The true test of whether kundalini has been raised is in the consistent character and noble behavior of an individual.

IS THE KUNDALINI DANGEROUS?

The Master answers:

"Is money dangerous? It is just an energy. Kundalini is a latent energy that can be used for total consciousness. The only dangerous thing is the person whose kundalini is raised properly. That person is totally conscious. He cannot be lied to or cheated or politically swayed. The kundalini is essential. As long as you practice a total discipline or a complete and balanced kriya, there is no difficulty. In Kundalini Yoga, you will notice that every meditaion and kriya has some form of mantra in it. This ensures the channelization of the energy."[3]

CREATIVE POTENTIAL

"**What is Kundalini?** The energy of the glandular system combines with the nervous system to become more sensitive so that the totality of the brain perceives signals and interprets them, so that the effect of the sequence of the cause becomes very clear to the man. In other words, man becomes totally, wholesomely aware. That is why it is called the Yoga of Awareness. As all rivers end up in the same ocean, all yoga ends up by raising the kundalini in the man. What is the kundalini? The creative potential of the man."[4]

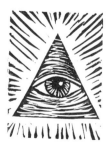

THE "DIVINE GLANDS"

PITUITARY

The pituitary gland, in addition to being the master gland of the body, also controls intuition. Sometimes called the "Third Eye," the sixth energy center of the body (Agia or Ajna Chakra) involves the pituitary gland.

PINEAL

The pineal gland is associated with the seventh energy center, the Shashara Chakra, sometimes called the "Thousand Petalled Lotus," "Tenth Gate," "Gate Of Salvation," or "Crown Chakra." (The soft spot on the top of a newborn baby's head, the fontanel, is at the 7th center.)

SCIENTIFIC, TECHNICAL INFORMATION
(Good to know)

PINEAL

The Pineal has several secretions that we in the West are just starting to learn about. Although, of course, the yogis have known its importance for thousands of years. One of the major functions of the pineal is to vibrate and control the nucleus projection of every cell of the body.

In most adults, the pineal gland is merely the size of a grain of wheat, while in young children it is about the size of a chick-pea. As most people get older, the pineal gland shrinks and its special secretion decreases. With the practice of Kundalini Yoga kriyas, the pineal gland can be softened, expanded and stimulated. It can grow to the size of an almond and begin again to secrete its consciousness-raising nectar. This special secretion is abundant in children.

CONSCIOUSNESS

All biological consciousness is chemical in nature. Our state of consciousness is controlled by the secretion of chemicals called neuro-humors, neurotransmitters, and blockers, in the various areas of the brain. "Raising the kundalini" causes the activation of certain chemicals in the brain through conscious and directed action.

BALANCE

In Kundalini Yoga, balance is extremely important. That is why we teach a total lifestyle, rather than just focusing on exercises to raise the kundalini energy. Everything we do in our lives affects our kundalini energy, and our kundalini energy affects everything we do in our lives.

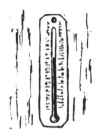

The vibrations of every word we speak, every thought we think, instantly raises or lowers our kundalini. It is as if we are registering our thoughts, moods, words, and actions on the most delicate and sensitive thermometer ever invented. It responds instantly to the slightest change in our vibration. Keeping the kundalini thermometer up requires monitoring every thought and word, otherwise, our vibration or frequency drops, or falls into the lower chakras. All the chakras are valuable, and we need to use all of them, but when the kundalini energy is primarily focused in our lower chakras, and we do not exercise any control over them, then we become slaves to our minds and emotions.

Without the consistency of maintaining a higher perspective by using the neutral mind, *(See Three Minds are Better Than One in Conquer the Mind)* there is seldom contentment. No matter what we achieve, what success in the world we have, it ends up being hollow unless we fulfill the soul's yearning to bring higher consciousness into our daily lives.

The essential nature of the soul is pure joy.
If I'm not experiencing joy,
then I'm not experiencing my soul.

8
Chakras
(Energy Centers)

"Where are you at?"

Until Yogi Bhajan taught what the chakras actually are, and how they influence our lives, I had no desire to explore the labyrinth of Sanskrit terms and esoteric symbology in the yoga books I had seen. The brilliantly colored lotus flowers, petals decorated with deities, animals or other symbols portraying the chakras were very pretty, but I didn't understand what connection they had to my life. Fortunately, what he has taught us about the chakras does not require any investigation into the occult. It's not myste-rious at all. On the contrary, the nature of the chakras and their functions is simple and to the point. The point being: wherever the majority of your kundalini energy is focused or polarized affects the way you are. The chakras do play a vital role in the way we human beings function, so let me go into a little detail and share with you the understanding the master of Kundalini Yoga has given us.

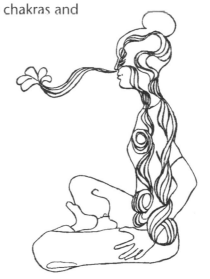

Chakras are centers of conscious-ness. They are focal points of energy which have a direct, immediate and profound effect on our daily lives.

THE ETERNAL FLOW OF POWER

Human beings have been designed by the Master Architect with patterns of energy flows. Energy flows through our spine, through our arms and legs and through eight specific energy centers, or chakras. Six of the projected centers of consciousness that correspond to these chakras are located in the body, while the seventh is just above the top of the skull, and the eighth chakra is the aura or magnetic field.

The energies of the first five chakras correspond to the five basic elements of which we are made: earth, water, fire, air, and ether.

WHERE ARE YOU AT?

The particular energy center or chakra, where the majority of your kundalini energy is primarily focused—or polarized—influences your basic behavior and attitudes. Let me make that even stronger, the chakra that you use as home-base for your kundalini energy pretty much determines the kind of person you are. The location of the major portion of your kundalini energy also accounts for the kinds of situations you attract to you.

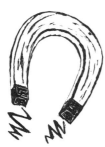

Just as in real estate, the three most important components are: location, location, location. Events become more understandable when we know where our energy is primarily located. Why? Because energy acts like a magnet. We constantly attract vibrations to ourselves that are on the same wavelength as the chakra from which we are operating. These vibrations are experienced as events and situations. People are drawn to us (not necessarily consciously) by the vibrations we project—knowingly or unknowingly.

Yes, it's also true that "opposites attract." Raising our kundalini to activate the neutral mind (sixth chakra) enables us to balance the forces of positive and negative that exist in every situation. Balance is one of the main keys to self-mastery and contentment. The yogi strives to achieve balance so that he is never thrown off base. In yogic terms it is said, "A yogi is not affected by the pairs of opposites." We practice Kundalini Yoga in order to balance and coordinate the functions of the lower chakras and to experience the realms of the higher chakras.

After the kundalini energy rises and becomes accustomed to flowing freely through all the chakras, there is a definite change of consciousness, a noticeable transformation in the character of an individual. The person looks at life differently, feels different and therefore acts differently. The real "proof" that someone's kundalini has risen lies in the upgrading of that person's attitude toward life, his relationships with other people, and with himself.

Raising the kundalini has to do with spiritual elevation. It is not to be confused with hearing sounds or seeing visions. When the kundalini is

Cherdhi Kalaa, **"high spirits" result when Kundalini returns down through Ida and Pingala and opens all the chakras!**

allowed to rise through the practice of Kundalini Yoga, it will not make a person weird or unbalanced. Note that the operative word here is "allowed." Kundalini Yoga does not force the kundalini to rise; it prepares the body to allow it to rise so that you can experience your higher consciousness. The object achieved is to coordinate and balance the functions of the chakras that are concerned with the needs of daily life with the universal consciousness and expansion that are found in the higher chakras. When this balance occurs, you become empowered, you are able to be a compassionate, conscious, and capable human being.

Some people think that merging with universal consciousness is a loss of identity. On the contrary, it is a loss of limitation. It is the discovery and experience of one's greater identity, which is infinite. Succinctly put, "Sat Nam: Truth is your identity."

THE EIGHT CHAKRAS

As my mother used to say, "There's a time and a place for everything." Each chakra has an important and necessary function to perform for us. We need all of them. No one chakra is better or worse than another, no chakra is more important than another. By understanding their purpose, we can make the best use of their power. The energy of the first five chakras corresponds to the five elements, Earth, Water, Fire, Air, and Ether. Think about the characteristics of these elements and you will have some clues as to the properties of the chakras associated with them.

FIRST CHAKRA: Earth

The first chakra represents the earth element in us. It is located in the rectum at the conjunction of 72,000 nerve endings. We couldn't get along without the first chakra. It enables us to eliminate solid waste, a most essential function of the physical body. The first chakra concerns have to do with the basic questions of security and survival. When functioning properly, this energy center gives a person strength and confidence. If it is not functioning properly, a person lives in fear and insecurity and can have a perverted approach to life.

SECOND CHAKRA: Water

The second projected center of consciousness has to do with the water element in our nature. It is located in the sex organs. When the second chakra is functioning properly, a person is creative and imaginative, energized and lively. Blockages in the second chakra can create an obsession with sex, to the point that nothing else matters in the person's life. There may also be an unhealthy indulgence in many kinds of fantasy, not only sexual fantasy.

THIRD CHAKRA: Fire

The third chakra represents the fire element in us. It is located in the navel point, a major focal point of energy where all 72,000 nerve endings meet. It controls the fire of digestion. The energy here is concerned with identity, domain, and judgment. If there is an imbalance, it can manifest in the person's character as excessive greed and an overwhelming drive for personal power. No matter how much a person gets, he always wants more. Nothing is ever enough, no matter whether it is needed or not.

As we do with the energy of all the chakras, we want to harness the energy of the third chakra so we can use it for our own benefit. On the positive side, third chakra energy gives us initiative and courage. Its fire can ignite a burning desire in us to accomplish great deeds and give us the zeal to keep up!

56

LOWER TRIANGLE MEETS HIGHER TRIANGLE

Although God can be realized through any one of the chakras, the first three chakras are designed mainly to deal with the physical needs and concerns of worldly life. It is the fourth chakra that is the balance point between these lower chakras and the higher chakras that are more concerned with universal consciousness.

FOURTH CHAKRA, or HEART CENTER: Air

The fourth projected center of consciousness is sometimes called the "Heart Center" or the "Center of Christ Consciousness." It is located at the center of the chest, not in the physical organ of the heart. The fourth chakra relates to the element of air in us. The power to sacrifice, born of universal divine love, comes from this chakra. It is the home of true maternal love.

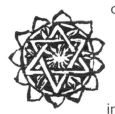

Any selfless act of giving without expectation of return comes from the heart center. It is the arena of kindness (the highest virtue) and compassion. When we truly speak "heart to heart" with someone, our language is sweet, kind, and uplifting, and the message gets across. When an awakened human being dwells in the fourth chakra, he is accessible, connected, loving, and compassionate.

Some people think of the heart center as the opening of feelings and emotions. Not true. Actually, it is the second chakra that opens sensory intensities, whereas the fourth chakra gives you a relationship to your feelings that changes commotion to devotion. It transforms passion to compassion. Coming from the heart center makes you act consciously about the whole range of feelings, it doesn't just intensify them.

❧   L O V E   ❧

We suffer a great deal in our lives because our kundalini energy is stuck in our lower three chakras (the lower triangle), most of the time. It is only when the heart chakra is stimulated and becomes active, that true love can be experienced.

What usually passes for "love" in our society is, at best, a business deal. It would be more accurately described as possessiveness or lust. "I'll love you if...." True love has no boundaries, no demands, and no limits. It is a total giving. Total acceptance. Love is blind, it doesn't question, and it doesn't find fault. Very few of us have ever experienced such true love, therefore we don't understand it. The saints and masters who have offered it to humanity have usually been crucified.

"To live is to love, to love is to give, to give is to have love." [1]

FIFTH CHAKRA, the THROAT CHAKRA: Ether

The fifth energy center has to do with the power and impact of speech. When we speak from the fifth chakra our words are direct and penetrating. They also may be painfully blunt. One of the primary characteristics of this fifth chakra is the power of projection. Anytime you succeed in penetrating with your words, the fifth chakra must operate. The fifth chakra commands by the word.

Being primarily focused at the throat chakra means we think about, talk about, are interested in nothing but Truth (i.e., God). However, when not functioning properly, the energy here can make us highly opinionated and what we communicate is our own personal limited version of "truth." The fifth chakra gives access to the arena of knowledge.

THE SIXTH CHAKRA: Intuition

The sixth chakra, or Ajna Chakra, located at the center of the forehead, slightly above the eyebrows, is sometimes called the "Third Eye."

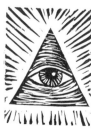

Here is where we can "see the unseen, know the unknown." It is from the sixth chakra that we gain access to, and increase our faculty of, intuition. The sixth chakra is the direct pipeline to the infinite source of universal knowledge and wisdom in each of us. When we function from the sixth chakra we can use our neutral or meditative mind; and tap into the knowledge of the past, the present, and the future.

58

As you focus more and more on the sixth chakra, your intuition becomes more active, and you will increasingly recognize and cherish breath, life, and intuition as gifts you have received.

The sixth chakra is the place to set your goals and assess the long-range effects of your actions. It is the arena of projection and sophistication.

The more we stimulate the pituitary gland via the sixth chakra, the more it will secrete, and the more powerfully intuition will serve us. We will just know!

Intuition is a higher faculty than intellect. It is in a different realm than the intellect. Nor is being intuitive the same as being psychic. Psychic power uses energy from, and functions through, the third chakra, not the sixth. Psychic abilities can be very useful, but psychic powers have many pitfalls. Being psychic is very individual and subjective, and there is a broad margin for error. Also, there can be a great temptation to use psychic power to control other people.

THE SEVENTH CHAKRA

Sometimes called the "Thousand Petalled Lotus," the seventh center of consciousness is at the top of the skull. It is also referred to as the "Gate of Salvation," "Tenth Gate," or "Crown Chakra."

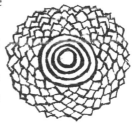

When a person raises and experiences the kundalini energy at the seventh chakra, he or she merges into a state of bliss (anand) that has been described as "indescribable." Hence the mantra of ecstasy, "Wahe Guru," which means "Wow! The experience of God is so fantastic, wonderful, and great I can't describe it!"

This state of divine union is known as "yoga" (sometimes referred to as samadhi). When a yogi leaves his body consciously to merge with the Infinite, it is through the seventh chakra. These are the enlightened beings. They teach us that "All things come from God and all things go to God."

EIGHTH CHAKRA: Aura

The Eighth Chakra is the magnetic field generated by the vibrations of a human being. Your aura surrounds you. It normally extends several feet in every direction. The quality and size of the aura reveals a lot about the person. It is either a projection of power or it can reveal the weakness and depression of defeat. This eighth chakra is your protective shield. It changes in color, strength, and size depending upon your general physical health, and your moment-to-moment thoughts and feelings. Many people are able to see the aura, many are 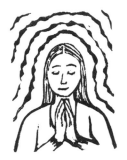 not — but it's there. Kirlian photography claims to capture the image of the aura on film. It is one of the many technical devices people have used to explore ways to register the changes in the aura and subtle body.[2] We may not see a person's aura, but we can feel it. We are often attracted or repelled by someone from our contact with their electromagnetic field.

BALANCE

Once the kundalini has risen up the central column of the spine and then returns down the ida and the pingala nerve channels to be distributed and balanced in all the chakras, a person's life takes on a new quality. Not too strong, and not too weak, but J U S T right (in perfect balance), is the way we want all of our chakras to function.

CHAKRAS, KUNDALINI, AND MY HAPPINESS

Where my kundalini energy is primarily focused affects how I am vibrating. Happiness does not live in low vibrations. It can't exist there. They are mutually exclusive. It's all a matter of vibration. It's not a matter of moral judgment. It's almost a mathematical equation: thoughts and words of kindness, compassion, generosity, love, sacrifice, etc, have a high frequency or vibration; whereas thoughts, words, and feelings of anger, jealousy, resentment, greed, egotism, fear, selfishness, etc. have a very low vibration. And so, of course, when we are involved in them, they pull us down to our lower chakras. It's almost like a piano keyboard. Whatever note you strike, that is what vibrates. When you hit middle "C," that is where you're at. (Secondarily, that tone vibrates all those notes that are in harmony with it, even on other octaves.) Your consciousness is exactly, precisely at that place, at any given moment, where your thoughts and words are vibrating.

NERVE OF THE SOUL

Yogi Bhajan speaks of the kundalini:

"Yes, kundalini is known as the nerve of the soul. This is to be awakened. Your soul is to be awakened. When soul gets awakened, there remains nothing. What else is there?

In the practical reality, these chakras are imaginary and nothing else. This kundalini is just a kundalini and nothing else. It is not very important. These pranas and apanas are just there. Everything is set in us. We lack nothing. We use these terms simply to make the process clear so we can get on with it. It is very simple. After getting myself into the darkness for years together, I found that if I would have known on the first day that it was so easy, I could have saved myself a lot of hassle. When I found out that the kundalini really can come up like this, I was astonished. It was a surprise to me. I said, 'That's all there is to the kundalini?' And my master said, 'Yes'!"

Now, I have to confess that the above quotation is incomplete. In the article quoted, he talks about prana and apana and the chakras, which he called "imaginary" (although they do exist). He's the master, and he has a way of putting things that is quite unique. He also says:

"All it is, creating the prana in the cavity and mixing it with apana and taking it down (as we give pressure to the oil) and bringing the oil up. This is kundalini. That's it. That is the greatest truth. Truth is bitter I know, so I cannot speak all the truth; but I speak indirectly and directly about the truth because I cannot speak something beyond truth..."[3]

TO SUMMARIZE:

You can improve your mood, lift your spirits, and brighten your day simply by raising your kundalini energy. We suffer when we let the first three chakras control us, instead of controlling and using their valuable energies for positive, constructive purposes. Each element has a positive and necessary function in our lives. Watch yourself. Are you starting to get angry? (You know that's bad for the digestive system!) Take a few long deep conscious breaths, bring your concentration up to your sixth chakra and with your neutral mind, decide, do you really want to lose your temper? That fire energy can be translated into enthusiasm, initiative, and courage. You can even choose to take third chakra energy and use it to run around the block. Do your cardio-vascular system some good. The point is to be able to choose and use, instead of living in self-abuse where you lose control.

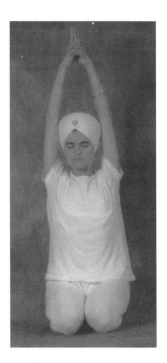

As you read the following chapters, and try the various sets of exercises, you'll be automatically using the energy of each chakra to work for you, not against you.

OKAY, you may be thinking, that all sounds very nice, but just exactly how do we raise the kundalini? It's simple: Go to the *Things To Do* section and learn to apply the Root Lock or Mul Bandh. Then practice Sat Kriya. Any exercise in which you apply the root lock helps to raise the kundalini. The root lock closes off the three lower chakras (the lower triangle) and therefore the kundalini energy must flow upward. It is like closing flood gates. There's nowhere to go but up!

Sat Kriya

9
Stress, Stamina
& Nerves of Steel

When I was a little girl back in Minnesota in the early thirties, appliances were built to last. I don't remember my mother ever buying a new toaster or a new iron. But periodically she would show us a frayed electric cord with the fabric wrapped around the cord worn so thin that the copper wires inside were exposed. She'd say it was time to get a new cord, because a frayed cord was dangerous. She explained that without insulation, bare wires could cause a short, blow a fuse or even start a fire!

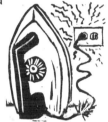

I can still picture those frayed cords, with their frazzled ends and the bare wires exposed. When I think about the nerves in our bodies, I see a network of 72,000 "wires" intertwining and connecting, carrying messages back and forth to the brain and throughout the nervous system. No matter how good our intentions, if our nerves are weak, frayed and frazzled, we can, and often do, blow a fuse. However, when our nerves are strong and well insulated, they give us physical and emotional endurance. Strong nerves make it possible for us to have patience. Otherwise, when our nerves are weak, we can fly off the handle at the slightest provocation and easily lose our tempers.

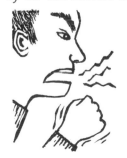

When anyone loses his temper, it means he has lost self control. Unfortunately, yelling and screaming in anger creates a false sense of personal power. That rush of adrenaline feels great—for the moment. But it doesn't last. When a person gets angry, the adrenals kick in to fuel the body's automatic defense system. The survival instinct of "fight or flight" triggers secretion of the adrenal glands.

63

Secreting large amounts of adrenaline not only overloads the adrenals, but taxes the pancreas as well. Those of us with weak adrenals and those who have hypoglycemia might just as well take poison as get angry! It has the same effect.

Self-control and common sense go out the window in a fit of anger. The rational mind stops functioning. People often say and do things they deeply regret later. Feelings can be hurt, and long-term relationships can be damaged or destroyed by careless words spoken in the heat of the moment.

Relationships crumble when you give anger a tumble.

Apologizing can never erase the imprint of the pain that was inflicted. People may forgive, but they usually don't forget. In fact, there is a permanent log of every word ever uttered. It is called the Akashic Record. It's not on paper, but it's there, just the same. Vibrations set in motion when we speak don't just disappear.

So, if you agree anger is damaging, does that mean that you should stifle your emotions? Grit your teeth, bite your tongue, and "stuff it" when you're provoked or aggravated? No. Not at all. Please read on. There's a better way to deal with frustrating situations.

THE FIRST STEP IS TO BUILD STRONG NERVES

Most of us want to be kind, relaxed, and loving people. We want to be wise and patient parents, understanding spouses, and good friends. But how can we be any of those things when every nerve is so raw it's shrieking in pain, and we're "on the edge," about to "lose it," most of the time?

STRESS

If our nerves are not strong enough to withstand the onslaught of life's daily challenges, then we are going to suffer from the number one killer disease of modern times: STRESS!

Every day brings some stressful situation, some test, big or small, which we have to face, to solve, to overcome. That's life, folks! Life is a school, and earth is a giant classroom and the tests are going to continue until we graduate. The outer events that occur, the daily challenges at home, in the office, the supermarket, on the freeway, are all tests. They are exercises in learning to master our minds and emotions so that we are not uptight and upset.

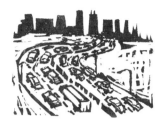

Learning how to be patient, calm, compassionate, and kind, no matter what happens around us, or to us, is not only a practical accomplishment. It's a yogic skill!

In California, we have earthquakes. As yet no one has figured out how to prevent them. No one can control them. It has been found that the main cause of injury is not the earthquake itself, but what happens when people panic. Instead of waiting calmly for the danger to subside, when panic takes over, people run madly about and get hit by falling debris, or electrocuted by live wires. We may not be able to change the circumstances happening around us, but we can learn to control the way we respond. And I don't mean by squelching or stifling our reactions or denying our emotions. Developing a strong meditative mind through Kundalini Yoga is a major step toward developing our own indomitable inner strength and serenity with the ability to call upon it whenever we need it.

ROBOTIC REACTION

Through meditation, mantra, and pranayam, we can tap into the absolutely calm and tranquil inner peace and stability that already exists inside us. With

> ### "Don't react—resurrect."
> —Yogi Bhajan

strong nerves and a balanced glandular system, we won't just "react" to situations. We will be in such a stable and secure mental and emotional condition

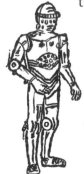

that whatever and whenever challenging events occur, we will be competent to evaluate our response and decide how we want to handle them.

As aware yogis, we can stop being reactive robots, and become calm and capable human beings, masters of our emotions and minds. Strong nerves play a big part in helping us to achieve all of the above.

65

THREE THINGS YOU CAN DO

• Breath of Fire is a powerful and rapid method of building strong nerves. Practice it every day.

• Breathe only through your left nostril for twenty-six long slow, deep breaths to calm yourself down in any tense situation.

• If you feel the heat of anger rising inside you, drink a full 8-ounces of water immediately.

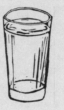

There may be times when you want to act forcefully, dynamically. There are times when you have to be assertive. That is different from being reactive. People who practice martial arts know they diminish their effectiveness if they get angry. They utilize the breath to center themselves. They inhale deeply before applying a karate chop or breaking cinder blocks with their bare hands. Remember, breath has atomic power. Use it wisely.

There may be times when it's useful to let people think you're angry. There may be times when it's required to yell and scream. But as for me personally, I have had to give up that "luxury" because just going through the motions of being angry, much less really feeling it, makes me physically ill. My system can't handle the adrenaline so I can't afford to be at the mercy of my emotions. I need to be able to choose intelligently when and where and how to respond to all situations. Besides, I don't want to be just a reactive machine, with buttons that anybody can push. I definitely don't want anybody to have that kind of control over me! How about you?

You do not have to let your emotions rule you. You can start by recognizing that your emotions are not you. Your emotions are not your identity! You can experience them and observe them happening at the same time, just as you will learn to observe your mind in action.

NERVES, MUSCLES, AND YOGA

Our nerves support our muscles and give us endurance. Endurance allows us to exercise longer and develop stronger muscles. When Yogi Bhajan was a young man in college in India, he was an all around athlete and track star. He played hockey and was captain of the soccer team. He says he used to train for athletic events primarily by doing yogic breathing exercises (pranayam). He knew yoga would give him the stamina and endurance to win the trophies. And win he did!.

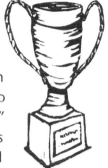

In the "Things To Do" section of this book, you'll find some exercises that are specifically for balancing your glandular system and strengthening your nerves. Will they really work? You'll have to practice them to find out. As we keep saying, "Doing is believing." For a fair trial, give yourself forty days of regular practice. It takes that long to develop a habit. It takes ninety days to confirm it, and after 120 days, others will verify it!

ANGER

Anger is a condition of frustration born out of the ego feeling powerless.

"The bold and handsome young Samurai warrior stood respectfully before the aged Zen master and asked, 'Master, teach me about Heaven and Hell.'[1] The master snapped his head up in disgust and said, 'Teach YOU about Heaven and Hell? Why, I doubt that you could even learn to keep your sword from rusting! You ignorant fool! How dare you suppose that you could understand anything I might care to say!' The old man went on and on, becoming even more insulting, while the young swordsman's surprise turned first to confusion and then to hot anger, rising by the minute.

"Master or no Master, who can insult a Samurai and live? At last, with teeth clenched and blood nearly boiling in fury, the warrior blindly drew his sword and prepared to end the old man's sharp tongue and life all in a moment. The master looked straight into his eyes and said, 'That's Hell.' At the peak of his rage, the Samurai realized that this was indeed his teaching; the Master had hounded him into a living Hell, driven by uncontrolled anger and ego.

"The young man, profoundly humbled, sheathed his sword and bowed low to his great spiritual teacher. Looking up into the aged wise man's beaming face, he felt more love and compassion than he had ever felt in his life, at which point the master raised his index finger as would a schoolteacher, and said, 'And that's Heaven.' "

10
Healing

Doctors diagnose, herbs & medicines cure, healing is a gift of God.

From time immemorial, there have been "healers," people who seem to have a special gift to ease pain, bring comfort, and cure others. Yet no person is really a healer — however, everyBODY can be a healer, including you and me.

Each of us can increase our ability to bring more healing energy to ourselves and to others. We can do this by tapping into the source of all healing power, the One Creator who breathes in each of us, regenerating us with each inhalation.

What does "healing" mean? Healing means bringing life to a situation or condition that is deteriorating. Healing means repairing, rejuvenating, regenerating.

Through the practice of Kundalini Yoga kriyas, breathing techniques, and mantras, we increase the life force, the prana, flowing through our bodies. It flows through our hands, our eyes, even our voice. We can use these as tools to heal ourselves and others.

Through the use of words vibrating in the form of mantra: positive affirmations and positive thinking, we can heal. Every word has its own wavelength, or frequency of vibration. Every word is a sound current (even if inaudible) which sets energy into motion. This energy goes out in ripples or waves and (to switch analogies in mid-ocean) the vibrations eventually return to us like a boomerang, bringing more of the same. There is power in positive thinking and positive affirmations! That power can work to expedite the healing process for ourselves and others.

SELF- HEALING

Do you believe it? Can you accept the fact that no matter what the outer circumstances in your life may appear to be, you have a right to be, Healthy, Happy and Holy?

Even if you're feeling lousy, especially if you are feeling lousy, and you're running a fever of 103 degrees; or you just broke your arm and lost your job, the truth is that there is a level of your being

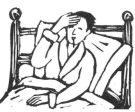

that is perfectly healthy, happy, and holy at all times.

SIMPLE SELF-HEALING MEDITATION

Sit (or lie down) with spine straight. Breathing only through the nose, inhale deeply then recite *aloud:*

HEALTHY AM I
HAPPY AM I
HOLY AM I

Inhale deeply again, feeling divine, loving, healing energy pouring into your body with each inhalation, and repeat the affirmation again. Continue for several minutes, taking in a deep breath between each cycle. Continue for as long as you choose. Do not be shy, chant loudly and forcefully so that the message sinks into your subconscious! Don't underestimate the power of this simple affirmation.

When you affirm (state and repeat) that you are "Healthy, Happy and Holy," you literally change your subconscious perception of what is happening. That perception accelerates the healing process.

We create whatever situation we affirm. Everything is "in the eye (or ear?) of the beholder." By mentally creating health, we set up favorable circumstances for that condition to manifest physically.

In the meantime, follow medical procedures. Don't throw away the prescription medicine yet, but understand (stand-under) and know that God is healing you rapidly, and keep telling yourself that you are now already vibrantly healthy! Positive affirmation is done in the present tense, because it is happening now in the sub-conscious.

How we view events and circumstances defines the impact they have on

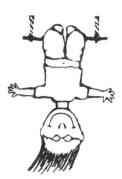

us! Using our convenient TV analogy, we can "switch channels" on our inner view screen from misery to comedy, from tears to laughter at any given moment. We each have that power. Try it, you may like it!

A mental condition can change instantly, the physical takes longer.

HEALING OTHERS

Everybody is a healer and nobody is a healer. There is only one true healer, sometimes called God, or God Consciousness. It is only through that One Divine Power that healing really takes place. Some people develop themselves to be especially clear conduits for it. Your very presence can heal others when your vibration reflects and projects the divine radiance of your soul.

Did you ever shake hands with someone whose touch felt so slimy, you couldn't wait to go and wash your hands? It's as If you'd been holding a dying fish. On the other hand (pardon the pun), did you ever shake hands with someone and feel the warmth of love, strength, and kindness flowing into you?

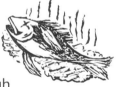

What you feel in both cases is the other person's electromagnetic field. His or her vibration is being transmitted to you. It is the vibrations people emanate that we feel, especially through touch. When a person is ill, their vibration lacks prana. We can, therefore influence someone else's condition by transmitting prana through our touch, our words, and our thoughts.

One of the interesting things about healing is that when we pray to heal someone else, we often heal ourselves. The way it works is that "What goes around, comes around." "As you sow, so shall you reap." The injunction to "Do unto others as you would have them do unto you," is a very practical guideline for life.The more we give, the more we shall receive.

ACROSS TIME AND SPACE
RAA MAA DAA SAA SAA SAY SO HUNG

Here is the most powerful healing vibration/mantra that I know. *(See facing page.)* It tremendously enhances your effectiveness as a "healer." Regular practice brings increased prana into your hands. For healing at a distance, this is the mantra. It cuts across time and space so you can send healing energy to someone thousands of miles away as easily as you can send it across the room. I have included the musical notation for the way I first learned it, with the instructions Yogi Bhajan gave for chanting it. (Later, he taught other variations of this melody.)

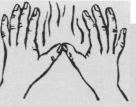

HEALING HANDS

Would you like to increase the kindness and effectiveness of your healing touch? Here's a simple routine you can practice that brings more prana into your hands.

1. Rub the palms of your hands together briskly for 3-5 minutes. Produce heat in the hands. Then stretch your arms out to the sides, parallel to the floor, palms up, thumbs pointing back. Breath of Fire for 3 minutes.

2. Then inhale, hold the breath in, and with the arms still out to the sides, bend your wrists, so your palms are facing out (away from the body) as if you were pushing out the walls on either side of you. FEEL THE ENERGY IN THE CENTER OF THE PALMS FLOWING TO YOUR ENTIRE BODY.

3. Rub hands together again for 2 minutes. Then, bend your left elbow, keeping the forearm parallel to the floor, with the left hand in front of the diaphragm, palm facing up, place your right palm facing down about 8 inches above the left palm. MEDITATE ON THE EXCHANGE OF ENERGY BETWEEN THE PALMS OF THE HANDS.

Practice this for 11 minutes every day if you want to be able to transfer healing energy to someone or some thing such as massage oil or a glass of water.

RAA MAA DAA SAA SAA SAY SO HUNG
TO SEND GOD'S HEALING POWER & ENERGY

To be chanted powerfully from the navel point for 11 minutes.
Sit in easy pose with the elbows tucked comfortably against your ribs. Extend forearms out at a 45 degree angle out from the center of the body. Palms are flat, facing up, fingers together, thumbs spread. Consciously keep the palms flat during the meditation. Be aware they may tend to curl up. Eyes are 9/10 closed.

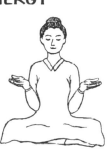

RAA	*Sun*
MAA	*Moon*
DAA	*Earth (Receiver of Totality)*
SAA	*Totality*
SAA	*Totality*
SAY	*Spirit, Energy*
SO	Manifestation
HUNG	*Experience of Thou*

Pull in the navel point powerfully on **SO** and **HUNG** and "clip off" each of these two syllables, making them short. Particularly note that HUNG is not long and drawn out. You clip it off forcefully as you pull in the navel.

Chant one complete cycle of the entire mantra, and then inhale deeply and repeat.

(Remember, chanting is not singing, it is vibrating.)

After 11 minutes, close your eyes, inhale deeply and hold the breath as you offer a healing prayer, visualizing the person you wish to heal as being totally healthy, radiant, and strong. Then exhale and inhale deeply again, hold the breath and offer your prayer..

You can do this several times, each time creating in your mind a picture of the person completely healed. You may want to imagine the person completely engulfed in healing white light.

To complete the meditation, inhale deeply, lift your arms up high and vigorously shake out your hands and fingers. Relax.

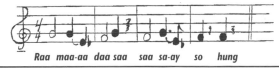

Raa maa-aa daa saa   saa sa-ay   so   hung

73

WORDS THAT HEALED—NOT!
The Power of Negative Thinking

Just to heal the physical body is not enough. *(See chapter on Ten Bodies.)* If we don't also heal the mental and emotional causes of a problem, it will most likely return in the same or some other form. That is why we emphasize the necessity for positive thinking and doing sadhana. *(For information on sadhana, personal spiritual practice, see Chapter on Sadhana.)*

Following is a true story. I know, because it happened to me.

It was one of those "cold" (for Los Angeles) rainy, winter days, and I was sitting on the floor of my old apartment on Preuss Road, doing bookkeeping for our newly formed 3HO Foundation. In the early 1970's I had no office so I worked at home. The financial department of 3HO consisted of some shoe boxes with receipts I kept in my closet. I held a full-time job at the Beverly Hilton, wrote letters for Yogi Bhajan, and handled the finances for his 3HO yoga classes in my spare time.

That historic day, I decided I could use a cup of hot tea to warm up. So I heated up the ever present pot of Yogi Tea on the stove and carried a steaming cup into the living room.

My feet felt cold, so I set the cup down carefully on the floor beside my books and papers, and went into the bedroom to put on a pair of socks. Talk about putting your foot into it! I came back into the living room, and forgetting the cup was there, I stepped right smack into the boiling hot tea. I let out a yell and ran to the bathroom. More accurately, I hopped on the other foot while clutching wildly at the sock, trying to tear it off as fast as I could, since of course the wet wool retained the heat of the liquid, and was burning furiously. I grabbed some ointment from the medicine cabinet and spread it on the injured foot, which already was turning a bright and angry red.

Yogi Bhajan had just come back to town from one of his teaching tours and I knew he was at Guru Ram Das Ashram, a half a block away. I picked up the phone and called him, assuming he would come running over immediately to comfort and heal me. Forget it!

When I told him what had happened, he said, "You'll be all right. I'm sending Pink Krishna (nicknamed for her rosy complexion, the happy result of months of eating only green vegetables) over to take care of you." And so he did. She arrived in just a few minutes, and helped set up a place for me to lie down on the couch. I knew I couldn't possibly sleep in my bed, and I didn't expect to sleep much anyway.

I phoned the Beverly Hilton, told the manager I had severely burned my foot, so I would not be able to come to work the next day. I lay down, closed my eyes and settled in for a restless night. I slept fitfully off and on, but lo and behold, when morning dawned, there was not the slightest trace of a burn. There was no discoloration of the skin and no pain. I was amazed and thrilled.

"You've got to Ac-Cent-U-Ate the Positive E-lim-in-ate the Negative and Latch on to the Affirmative. Don't mess with Mr. Inbetween..."
—Hit Song by Johnny Mercer, circa 1940

I called my mother and said, "Guess what happened..." I told her the whole story of the hot tea, the burning sock, the amazing healing, and finished by saying "I don't believe it!" I called at least four other people and repeated the story, each time ending with the words, "I don't believe it!" By four o'clock in the afternoon my foot didn't believe it either. It started to ache and burn again. The redness returned in full force and I spent several weeks waiting for the slow process of nature to heal my foot. I learned that day about the power of my words!

We do create with every word we speak, and the power of positive (or negative) thinking and speaking is not a fantasy, it's a reality.

I had a different opportunity to experience the power of my words many years later when I slipped and fell down a flight of cement steps early one morning and broke two ribs. One of the advantages of breaking ribs is that they heal themselves back together perfectly, (and people are very kind to you while you're recuperating). However, in the meantime, you can't laugh or cough or even take a deep breath without severe pain. The pain, in spite of medication, could be quite intense, so I decided to try some of the yogic technology I had been preaching. And, I discovered, "By George, it works!" Whenever I felt a major twinge of pain, I'd say out loud (or just think), "Thank you God, I accept your wonderful gift of pain," and it would ease up immediately.

Gratefully accepting everything that comes to us as a gift of God invokes a remarkably dynamic response from God. An "attitude of gratitude" invites and allows the power of God to work faster and easier to bless and heal us.

Try it for yourself. Whenever anything happens — good, bad, pleasant, unpleasant, desirable, undesirable — see it as something that God is doing. Then verbally express and affirm your gratitude. See what happens. At least have the faith to try it as an experiment. Even if someone does something lousy, thank God that it's not you doing it! The person doing the lousy thing has that lousy karma to deal with. How you respond becomes your karma.

GURU RAM DAS TO THE RESCUE

At one point in his life, when Yogi Bhajan was threatened and harassed by people trying to do him harm, he meditated and prayed, calling on Guru Ram Das for help, and Guru Ram Das gave him this special mantra to use whenever he — or anyone — is in danger. (You can use it, too.)

GURU GURU WAHE GURU, GURU RAM DAS GURU

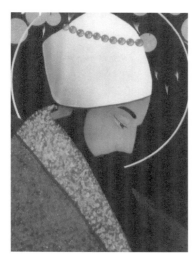

When we chant to Guru Ram Das, we are not chanting to a person, but rather to the consciousness that he embodied, and we are invoking the special qualities that he represented. "Ram" in itself is one of the Hindu names of God, and "Das" means servant. Ram Das was indeed, a beloved servant of God. He was a Raj Yogi and the fourth in the line of Sikh Gurus. Each of the ten Gurus personified and exemplified special virtues, and manifested certain qualities, to demonstrate that a person in any walk of life can be divine. Loved and respected for his humility, service, and compassion, Guru Ram Das was also a great Yogi, especially renowned for his extraordinary gift of healing.

HAIL GURU RAM DAS
and HEAL THE WORLD !

What you are about to read is a true story. No names have been changed. This really happened.

In 1938, when Yogi Bhajan was nine years old, he contracted a serious ear infection. Neither his father, who was a physician, nor any of the doctors and healers consulted, could find a way to cure it and the infection was spreading. He was diagnosed as incurable. He was expected to die.

During his sleep one night, the young boy had a visit from Guru Ram Das who told him that he should ask his father (Dr. Kartar Singh Puri) to put some onion juice in the infected ear. He told his father of the strange request. Sure enough, the treatment worked!

From that time onward, Harbhajan Singh Puri, later to become Yogi Bhajan, looked upon Guru Ram Das as his special protector, teacher, and guide. 3HO Ashrams around the world are named in honor of the great soul of Guru Ram Das.

Guru Ram Das was a "Raj Yogi." The famous Golden Temple in Amritsar, India, was built in his honor. It is called Hari Mandir Sahib and is

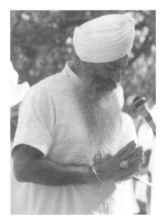

considered the holiest of holy places by Sikhs all over the world. Open to people of all religions, all colors, all nationalities, it is a sacred shrine where tens of thousands of people come to be inspired and uplifted by the vibrations of the Guru, and to sip and dip in the healing waters surrounding the Temple. Hari Mandir Sahib is built half of marble and half of gold.

As a young man, Yogi Bhajan washed the marble floors of the Golden Temple every night for four years, to cleanse and purify himself — praying to Guru Ram Das. He went in as a yogi and came out a saint. Such is the power and majesty of Guru Ram Das.

BRIEF LESSON IN HISTORY OF THE SIKH GURUS

Of the ten Sikh Gurus, one was a very young child, several were very old men, some were married, some were single. Some were poets, some were soldiers. Guru Ram Das, who lived from 1534 to 1581, was the fourth Guru to carry the divine light and infinite consciousness of Guru Nanak, the first Guru. Guru Nanak taught that everyone is inherently divine, and that people should not fight about how to worship the One God who breathes in everybody. His followers, or students were called "shishyas," or "Sikhs." Sikhs no longer worship any person as Guru, but look to the Siri Guru Granth Sahib, the embodiment of the Word of God (Shabd Guru), as their living Guru.

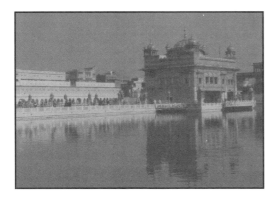

78

CHAPTER 11 • LET'S TALK ABOUT FOOD

11
Let's Talk About Food

Here are some clichés that are true (clichés often are):

- **You are what you eat.**
- **Your body is the living temple of God.**
- **Eat to live, don't live to eat.**

For thousands of people, controlling their diet is one of life's biggest challenges. It's a daily battle of will power versus compulsion and habit. Health clubs, gyms, and spas are overflowing with bodies stretching and straining, huffing and puffing, grunting and sweating to "get rid of ugly, unwanted body fat" and achieve ideal body weight. Fat or thin, we can be badly undernourished, if we're not getting the foods our bodies need.

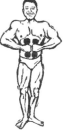

Dining on expensive gourmet food smothered in rich gravies and exotic sauces seems to be considered a sign of "success" in our society. Of course ulcers, gastritis, constipation, and overweight, not to mention high blood pressure and heart disease, can result from overeating or eating the wrong foods (and you don't have to be rich to gorge on foods way too high in fat content or salt). Overweight is not only damaging physically but psychologically.

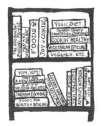

Dozens of different books promoting dozens of different diets are spilling over the bookstore shelves. Television ads

79

Kundalini Yoga: The Flow of Eternal Power

abound with weight-loss programs. Each one claims to have the perfect solution. However, being able to apply any solution requires a change in our habits, including our habitual way of thinking about ourselves. Fortunately, the yogis have given us methods to help us change our habit patterns. (*Please read the chapter called Creatures of Habit, and refer to the "Meditation to Change Habit Patterns).* Meanwhile, let's talk about food.

LIVING TO EAT or EATING TO LIVE?

There are two kinds of eating. The first kind is what is called recreational eating. This is eating purely (actually not purely) for taste or to be sociable. Recreational eating often consists of junk food. What do I mean by junk food? Any substance that leaves an excess of toxic waste in the body that you can't eliminate within twenty-four hours. Any food that depletes the body of vitamins, overstimulates the nerves, or overtaxes the pancreas is junk food in my book!

The second kind of eating is the kind of eating that nourishes, sustains, and energizes the body. It's known as "eating to live." We spend a large portion of our lives eating. What and how we eat affects us physically, mentally, and emotionally. Let's talk about eating from the standpoint of the yogis, whose purpose is to get the best out of every aspect of life.

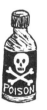

Let me share with you some yogic information, keeping in mind that each of us is different and has individual dietary requirements. One man's meat really is another man's poison. Each of us needs to find the right balance, the chemical combination of foods that best serves our metabolism and bodily needs. Meals should look appetizing and taste good, too. Healthy food doesn't have to be dull and boring or taste like straw. Eating a healthy diet does not have to be distasteful.

TO EAT OR NOT TO EAT?

In ancient books of knowledge, the Vedas, we can find instructions on how to eat, such as, "never eat to full stomach." Only one-half of the stomach's capacity is to be used for solid food, leaving one-quarter for liquid and the remaining one-quarter left empty to allow the digestive process to take place more easily.

It is also recommended to leave a gap of four to five hours between meals for the same reason. Otherwise, the blood is kept so busy working in the digestive area that other parts of the body are cheated out of their blood supply. The eyes, ears, nose, and throat particularly need good circulation. When these areas are weak and undernourished because of poor circulation, they are vulnerable to attack from bacteria and viruses that cause colds, flu, and infections. If you need to eat more often, okay, but you don't have to eat a lot. Try a light snack when your blood sugar gets low.

A person with a hypoglycemic condition whose blood sugar level fluctuates wildly because the pancreas is not able to do its job correctly, usually needs to eat something every two hours. Do read Dr. Paavo Airola's book *Hypoglycemia, A Better Approach*. You'd also be wise to read the book called *Sugar Blues* by Duffy.

You may be served the best, most delicious meal in the world, but, as my mother used to say, if it doesn't "agree with you," if you can't digest and eliminate it properly, it's probably doing more harm than good. Food is supposed to give us energy. It's supposed to be fuel for the body, feed the cells, and be transformed into blood, bones, and tissue. Whatever we eat that is not used for these purposes becomes waste matter, and needs to be eliminated. If the body cannot eliminate it fast enough, it becomes toxic and we get sick. We have literally poisoned ourselves. Whatever we eat should be digested and assimilated within 18 hours for a female and 24 hours for a male.

CHEW, CHEW, CHEW!
You don't have teeth in your stomach!

There's a way to tell if you're digesting your food properly or not, which could be called the "float test." If most of what you eat is being correctly utilized by the body, and is serving to heal and nourish, then what is left over as roughage will be minimal, and when you eliminate, it will float. If your stool sinks to the bottom of the toilet, then you can bet you have not gotten much real value out of your food intake.

A major factor in proper digestion takes place in your mouth. Food has to be well chewed so the digestive enzymes in the saliva can mix thoroughly with it. If you gobble your food in a hurry, you miss the crucial first step in the digestive process. Then when the food reaches the stomach, it's not prepared for proper digestion to take place. Take your time eating. Try counting twenty to fifty chews per mouthful—it will really slow you down. Another tip, if you're trying to cut down on portions: wait about five minutes before taking seconds on anything. Usually that waiting period is enough for the body to recognize it really has had enough. Otherwise, when you're eating too fast, you often keep on eating when you're not actually hungry any more.

WATER, WATER, EVERYWHERE
(You Need More Than A Drop To Drink)

Another clue to good digestion: Drink lots and lots of water, but don't wash down your food by drinking any liquid immediately after you take a bite of food. Washing down your food dilutes the enzymes that are needed for proper digestion. Do your kidneys a favor, start your day with two glasses of water after you brush your teeth. *(See Chapter on How to Get Up in the Morning.)* Keep a pitcher of water on your desk at work, and drink water all day. Eight glasses a day aren't even enough—try for sixteen—or at least twelve. At night, just before bed, drink a glass of water. You can monitor the health of your kidneys by observing the color of your urine first thing in the morning. It should be lighter than gold. If it is darker, you're in trouble. Drink more water. Maybe it's time to get a medical check-up.

EAT TO LIVE

Okay, so what is a healthy yogic diet? Well, for one thing, it's not fanatic, or weird, or tasteless. It is a balanced combination of:

- fruits
- nuts
- vegetables
- grains
- legumes
- dairy products

Despite what most airlines think, many vegetarians do eat dairy products although we don't eat eggs. When you practice Kundalini Yoga with Breath of Fire, it tends to eliminate mucous. Therefore, you want to replenish the system with a certain amount of mucous which dairy products can stimulate. Mucous keeps the breathing passages lubricated and protects the membranes. If you are allergic to cow products, then try soy or goat substitutes. Everyone is different, you have to find what works for you.

You may have noticed that meat, fish, poultry, and eggs are not on our list of foods. You are correct. Yogis don't eat them. You don't need them. You can get all the proteins, vitamins, and minerals you need from other foods. We do our arteries a big favor by avoiding foods that clog them up. A yogic diet is a vegetarian diet. There are excellent reasons for this. Here are three of them.

THREE EXCELLENT REASONS TO EAT A VEGETARIAN DIET

EXCELLENT REASON # 1

When we eat meat we're feeding ourselves the poisonous adrenaline that was secreted by the terrified animal just before it was slaughtered.

EXCELLENT REASON # 2

If it could ever walk, run, crawl, swim, or fly away, I don't want it on my plate!

Lions and tigers and other carnivores (whom God obviously intended to eat other animals, to keep the balance of nature) are provided with fangs, claws, and a very short intestinal tract. They can process flesh very quickly and eliminate it before it putrifies and becomes toxic. Our digestive tract is very long, so we can't.

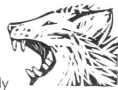

If you're worried about being weak without eating meat, think about the elephant. This great and powerful beast who feeds only on plants — lives very long, and is extremely intelligent.

EXCELLENT REASON # 3

Meat will leave a residue of uric acid in the bloodstream. Uric acid is considered by some to be a carcinogen (cause of cancer). Uric acid is a toxin that makes it harder to reach the higher, clearer meditative states because it is an irritant in the bloodstream.

COMMON SENSE

Ancient yogic teachings prohibit the eating of flesh and of anything that is burnt, stale, or decayed. Food that is simple, wholesome, fresh, and as natural as possible is recommended.

POOR FISH !

What about fish? You've heard the expression, "poor fish!" Caught by a cruel hook in its mouth, when it is dragged painfully out of its home in the ocean, river, lake, or stream, it dies an agonizing death deprived of water. If fish is not put into water or ice immediately, it begins to decay and stink. Even after it is eaten, it still demands water. Notice how thirsty you get after eating fish? It is still demanding water. Eating fish dehydrates the body. That sagging flesh under the upper arms can be traced to eating fish. Any questions?

EGGS: YOU HAVE TO DECIDE

Okay, let's talk about eggs. Setting aside any discussion about the living or dead aspect of the potential chicken in each egg, there is a very high cholesterol level in eggs. If you want to be kind to your arteries, whether you're a yogi or not, you don't eat eggs.

THROW OUT THE STEAK?

Good grief! No meat, no fish, no chicken (that's right, no fowl either), no eggs, what am I going to eat?

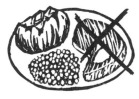

A vegetarian diet does not mean to take a plate with a steak, a baked potato, and a serving of peas and throw away the steak. Nor does it mean to fill up on pasta and bread. There is a vast assortment of delicious food growing in the ground, on trees, plants, and vines to choose from. And you don't have to live on a farm to get them. Health food stores and supermarkets almost everywhere carry plenty of things that are good and good for you. Augmented with marvelous herbs and spices which add flavor and are healing as well, vegetarian meals can be glorious experiences. By following an intelligent well-balanced vegetarian diet, you can live longer, be more energetic, and even sleep better. The Hunzas are said to live longer than any other group of people in the world, and they are vegetarians.

We shouldn't forget that we live on prana. We need to get prana from the food we eat and the water we drink as well as the air we breathe. Some foods give us more prana than others, depending upon their quality and condition.

In the recipe section of this book you'll find a few of my favorite recipes that even your non-vegetarian family and friends will enjoy. I've also listed the cookbooks I personally recommend to help you discover some creative and delicious meals you can make that will be kind to your body and satisfy your appetite.

For more information on meat eating, please refer to Diet For a New America by John Robbins and What's Wrong With Eating Meat? by Barbara Parham.

MUNG BEANS AND RICE ARE NICE

One of the most nourishing and easiest to digest foods is a dish called Kitcheree. It's a traditional Indian recipe made of mung beans and white basmati rice. Polished rice is not recommended because it has been stripped of its beneficial vitamin content. Brown rice is not recommended either, because it is very hard to digest unless it is cooked for many, many hours.

The mung bean is a tiny, humble little bean, dark green in color. It packs a lot of energy, and is high in protein. A basic recipe for kitcheree is in the recipe section of this book. You can vary it quite a bit to suit your own taste and creativity. One of the best things about kitcheree, besides the fact that it tastes so good, is that it contains four of the most important basic yogic foods for healing. Read on...

THE BIG FOUR: "HERB ROOT TRINITY" PLUS ONE

Onions, garlic, and ginger, often called the Herb Root Trinity, work together to cleanse the body and produce and maintain energy. The beneficial effect of each of them separately is amplified when they are cooked together.

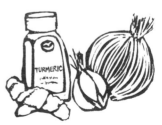

GARLIC

You may have heard that some ascetics will not eat garlic because it makes them more sexually potent . Garlic does help produce more semen (powerful creative energy) in the body. This increased sexual energy is controlled and moreover utilized by the practice of Kundalini Yoga. So we are not afraid of it. On the contrary, we want to increase it so we can channel it upward for greater spiritual awareness.

Considered a sacred herb by the ancients, for its powerful therapeutic effect, garlic oil has been found to battle effectively against many types of virus and bacteria. Garlic and garlic extracts have been used against gastrointestinal disorders, septic poisoning, typhus, and even cholera. In fact, Garlic was known in the former Soviet Union as "Russian Penicillin"!

Best eaten raw, garlic can also be taken in capsule form (in case your friends don't share your enthusiasm for this fragrant herb). You can make a very palatable spread for toast or crackers with finely chopped raw garlic mashed into avocado. A whole bulb of baked garlic is delicious spread over toast. You just squeeze out the individual cloves, after it's baked. Very gourmet! Garlic is most at home cooked in combination with onions and ginger.

ONIONS

The onion has a well earned reputation for being a universal healing food. It not only attacks harmful bacteria and purifies the blood, but it helps build new blood. It has been recommended for such things as colds, fever, laryngitis, and diarrhea (drink onion juice mixed with hot or cold mint tea). And it has even been said, "An onion a day keeps the cancer away." If you're going to travel to any foreign country where your body will have to deal with strange and unfamiliar bacteria, eating one raw onion every day for a couple of weeks before your trip, as well as while you're away from home, will help you avoid dysentery. If you can't handle eating onions raw, at least eat them cooked. Get them into your system somehow. There is even the claim that eating raw onions helps mental clarity.

GINGER ROOT

Ginger root is both soothing and strengthening to the nerves when the body is under stress. It helps strengthen the nerve centers in the spine by nourishing the cerebrospinal fluid. You can make a delicious and revitalizing tea out of ginger root very easily. Just slice an inch or two of ginger root (available in most grocery stores, supermarkets, and of course in health food stores) and boil it in a quart of water for a few minutes. For this recipe you don't even have to peel the ginger. Just strain the tea after it has boiled for a while, and it's ready to drink. You can add sweetener and/or milk if you wish. Ginger tea is particularly useful for women to drink during menstruation. It is great as a "pick-me-up" if you're feeling droopy and debilitated. Try it. It strengthens the nerves instead of destroying them the way caffeine does.

TURMERIC

Good for the skin and mucuous membranes, especially the female reproductive organs, turmeric is one of the main ingredients in curry powder. It adds flavor and can be used in many recipes, casseroles, soups, gravies, and sauces. It's a standard ingredient in Kitcheree. The virtues of turmeric have been lavishly praised by Yogi Bhajan. One of its most important properties is that it makes the bones and joints more flexible. Just a small amount has a positive effect. See the recipe section for Golden Milk, a great beverage for you and your children. Turmeric is on the spice shelf of your supermarket. Warning: be careful not to spill it on your clothes when you're cooking, because it stains when it's wet.

Kundalini Yoga teachings recommend eating the herb root trinity, garlic, onion, and ginger daily. Also, it's a good idea to get some turmeric in you (not on you) every day and drink at least one cup of:

YOGI TEA

This section would not be complete (and as it is, it's only a tiny peek at the vast amount of information and technology available about food. *The Ancient Art of Self Healing* by Yogi Bhajan describes many more yogic uses of food), without a major mention of Yogi Bhajan's famous YOGI TEA recipe. Yes, it's available now commercially, in bulk or in tea bags. In 1969 Yogi Bhajan taught me how to make it from scratch. He told me how he used Yogi Tea when he was out in the field, commanding a battalion of the Indian Army. A

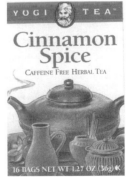

serious epidemic of flu broke out so all the troops were being sent home from maneuvers. However, he kept his men healthy and they stayed on duty because he had them fill their thermos bottles with Yogi Tea and drink nothing else, not even water. None of them got sick.

This amazing beverage is a standard item in the 3HO way of life. If you'd like to make it from scratch, you'll find his original copyrighted recipe in this book. The fun part of making your own Yogi Tea using the different spices, as Yogi Bhajan taught me, is that after the water comes to a boil, you add the cloves first and "watch them dance." Sure enough, they pair off, and dance around in groups of twos and threes! Then, in a minute or two, when the cloves have surrendered their essence to the water, that's when you add the other ingredients.

The black pepper is to purify the bloodstream, the milk is to soothe the colon so the black pepper doesn't irritate it. The cinnamon is for the bones, cardamom for the colon, and cloves for the nervous system. The ginger root is optional, but is highly recommended. If you want to clean out your system, you can go on a Yogi Tea fast. For one or two days—maximum three days— live on Yogi Tea. Drink as much as you want, and don't eat anything else. See how light and energetic you feel.

At least one cup of Yogi Tea per day is a great idea. Yogi Tea is more than a recipe for a good tasting drink, it is a formula for a complete self-healing tonic! Don't omit the black tea; it's part of the formula. These days, Yogi Tea also comes commercially packaged in various flavors. Ah, modern technology.

HIDDEN INGREDIENT

A most healing and effective ingredient in the food you cook, especially if you're a woman, is the VIBRATION you put into it. This is for real. It's not imaginary. When you pray and chant over food while you cook it, you enhance its power to nourish and heal.

Let me tell you a true story about vibrations going into food. A number of years ago a young woman came to stay at the 3HO center in Los Angeles to sort out her marital problems and get her life on track. She was an excellent cook, and she would prepare meals for several staff members every day. The food tasted delicious, but every afternoon after lunch we all felt sick. Finally we figured out that she was so angry all the time that it was affecting the food she cooked. We stopped eating her cooking until she came back the next year. Then, since she was in much better shape emotionally, we found we could enjoy her meals without getting sick. *(Much more on the subject of the extra power of women in the chapter on women.)*

Speaking of cooking, I used to worry and agonize over having to prepare meals for anyone, especially unexpected guests. I was never confident that they'd like what I made. What Yogi Bhajan taught me about cooking was to "use whatever you have, and chant while you prepare the food."

Vibration really makes a difference. And, of course, Yogi Bhajan is a fabulous cook. Many of his personal recipes were used in the Golden Temple Conscious Cookery Restaurants throughout the world and are included in the cook book he wrote. *(See the Cookbook section of the book list.)*

FOODS THAT LIKE YOU

A word in praise of zucchini. It's sooooooo easy to digest, hardly seems to have any calories, and is really fast to cook. You can slice it or not and simply steam it, or you can sauté it with onions and garlic and even put tomato sauce over it.

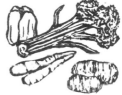

Use lots and lots of green vegetables in your diet. Use foods that are filled with prana (life energy), such as ripe, juicy fruits and almost anything that is in season and fresh. Ideally eat fresh rather than frozen foods, and frozen rather than canned. You can squeeze lemon juice on vegetables instead of using salt. There are many salt substitutes on the market made from a combination of herbs. The yogis say to avoid salt after age thirty-five. Read labels when you buy products. Avoid MSG and other chemicals. As much as possible use foods in their natural state, in other words, the less processing the better.

HOW SWEET IT IS!

We are a sweet nation. Americans consume tons of sugar annually. Sugar depletes the system of Vitamin B. Personally, I have found, my body and my nervous system cannot tolerate white sugar. It makes me very short-tempered. If I lose my temper, I blow out my adrenals and then I get sick. It has happened enough times for me to be sure of the sequence of events, and the consequences I suffer. There are plenty of ways to avoid sugar if you're serious about it. For one thing, taste can be conditioned.

I try not to add any sweetener at all to my Yogi Tea or other beverages. There are other things to eat that can appease the desire for sweets, and that craving diminishes when you're eating enough of the good stuff that your body needs.

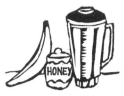

Applesauce cooked with cinnamon in it tastes lovely. You can use vanilla for flavor in yogurt or milk shakes. I like to put a frozen banana in the blender with milk (I use soy milk), a pinch of cinnamon, and a dash of vanilla. It can be made thick like frozen yogurt to eat with a spoon, or thinner like a shake — tastes great. For baking, maple syrup, maple sugar, or barley malt sweetener are available. Honey, although a very pure food, unfortunately is so concentrated that it can be hard on the pancreas. Some people do fine with fructose, whereas some people do not. Watch out for aspertaine. It's been reported to produce unwelcome side-effects.

Did you ever notice how "hyper" children get after they have eaten the sugar candy, ice cream, or cake treats we give them? One thing I know for sure, refined white sugar causes me to suffer, so I simply don't eat it. I can vouch for the difference in my life, health, and behavior since I stopped eating sugar. Read labels carefully and proceed accordingly. Sugar can be hidden in unexpected places.

WARNING: ALL CHOCOLATE LOVERS: DO NOT READ THE NEXT SECTION. YOU WON'T LIKE IT.

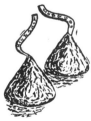

CHOCOLATE

Chocolate contains caffeine and theobromine. It is addictive. If you must have chocolate, at least try to get it sweetened with something other than white sugar. Sugar and chocolate seem to form a lethal combination. More and more people are becoming aware of the detrimental effects of sugar and chocolate, and there are a number of alternative products on the market. Check them out. You may actually like them, and they may like you, too!

The Surgeon General of the United States issues warnings saying that smoking causes cancer, but still, people smoke. So I don't expect my readers will give up their chocolate habits very easily. Some of us have weaned ourselves from

90

chocolate by training the taste buds to enjoy carob. Some people can tolerate chocolate when it's sweetened with honey or maple syrup, but personally, I don't want to get hooked on the taste of chocolate in any form. One of the key impacts of chocolate is that it stimulates neurochemicals in us that are cortical mood alterers. It produces feelings of connection and intimacy. No wonder chocolate is addictive! When you need consolation and comfort, you might try talking to your soul, it's the greatest chocolate kiss!

CAFFEINE

Caffeine depletes the pranas, and do I really have to say anything about what caffeine does to the nervous system? A yogi usually avoids all stimulants. 'Nuff said.

ALCOHOL

For rubbing, if you need to take down a fever, alcohol can be useful. As a beverage, it acts as a stimulant — at first — and then a depressant. It causes the liver to deteriorate and damages the brain. Alcoholics Anonymous can give you plenty of information about alcohol as an addiction.

YOU SAY YOU ATE A ROCK?

If, perchance, by mistake you eat too much (we Americans tend to stuff ourselves at every opportunity, eating too much and too often), there's a way to get some relief from that overstuffed feeling. Try sitting on your heels for a few minutes. Probably best not to do this in public, unless you want to attract a crowd. But if you're at home, sit in rock pose, Vajar Asan, for a few minutes after dinner. It is said that one can digest rocks by sitting in this posture. Or, for meditation it's supposed to help you sit steady as a rock.

SELF-HEALING KRIYA FOR DIGESTION

In my youth, out of ignorance, I foolishly tried some very fanatic experiments with fasting. They left me with serious digestive problems. My digestive system was so bad that when I met Yogi Bhajan, I couldn't even drink a glass of water without suffering. He taught me Vatskar Dhouti Kriya, and told me to do it for forty days, without missing a day. It helped me tremendously. Want to try it yourself? Turn the page...

VATSKAR DHOUTI KRIYA
To Master the Digestive System

This is one of the secret kriyas in Kundalini Yoga that for centuries had been taught only to the selected few. It is surprisingly simple and quite easy to do, but I assure you it works.

(Warning: Don't do this Kriya if you've just eaten, because it has to be done on an empty stomach.)

Sit in any posture with the spine straight. Make your lips round, in an "O" shape, and start inhaling the air as if you're drinking it in a series of repeated small sips. Inhale as many sips as you can possibly hold and then stop, close your mouth, hold the breath in and rotate your belly, churning your stomach with your breath held in until you can't hold the breath any more. Then very, very slowly and gently release the breath in one stream through the nose. Repeat this cycle again, inhaling in sips, holding the breath and churning the stomach then exhaling through the nose for a total of three cycles. This constitutes one complete kriya. According to yogic teachings, you are prohibited from practicing Vatskar Dhouti Kriya more than twice in any one day.

Note that in this kriya you are inhaling through the mouth which is an exception to the general rule of always breathing through the nose. If you want to gain control of your digestive system, practice Vatskar Dhouti Kriya once or twice a day for forty days. Don't miss a day.

MAKING A TRANSITION

I became a vegetarian in 1956, when it was suggested to me that if I stopped eating meat, my health would improve. I did, and it did. One approach to vegetarianism is to slowly and gradually substitute meatless main dishes in your meals and start eating more fresh fruits and vegetables. You could try being a vegetarian for one or two days a week at first, then gradually increase the number of days. Or there's the "cold turkey" (no pun intended) approach, such as the transition diet Yogi Bhajan gave in 1969. That diet consisted of thirty days of eating just fruits, nuts, and vegetables. Many of the students who went on it reported feeling kind of weak for the first few days, but they said after that the energy level picked up amazingly. After thirty days you add grains and dairy back into the picture, and, congratulations, you have made a graceful transition to a vegetarian diet!

THANKSGIVING

At least one day in the year, most Americans remind themselves to be grateful for the bounty we receive from the Creator. Blessed are those who give thanks every day, with every breath.

> **"Vegetarians don't eat anything that had a mother."**
>
> —Yogi Bhajan

Giving thanks before we eat anything, asking the real Giver of the food to bless it, is a very valuable habit. Blessing food adds prana to it. Prayers don't always have to be eloquent and lofty. I've heard Yogi Bhajan say things like, "Thanks a lot, God, we were really hungry and you gave us food. Please bless it and bless us. Thanks."

SUMMARY

To conclude this chapter, I suggest that you decide what you would like to incorporate or change in your existing pattern of eating. In any lifestyle change, it's important to be moderate and sensible rather than fanatic. If you've always been a big meat eater, don't try to become a vegetarian overnight. On the other hand, some people have successfully done it just that way. Use your own best judgment and common sense. And remember to:

- **Chew every mouthful of food thoroughly.**
- **Drink lots of water.**
- **Don't eat too often, don't eat too much.**
- **Laugh a lot.**

YOU ARE WHAT YOU EAT!

Tigers have fangs and long sharp claws
If they devour a deer or a lamb, they're obeying natural laws
All carnivores whom God intended to be
Have short intestinal tracts —Not long ones, like you and me.

Whatever we eat has to take a circuitous route
We're much better off with vegetables and fruit,
Nuts and berries, grains, milk, and cheese
Vegetarian diet designed to please.

If it walks, swims, or crawls
A vegetarian doesn't eat it at all
Elephants live long and carry plenty of weight
You won't find a steak on an elephant's plate.

Whatever you eat, make sure it digests
What's not used by the body
Must be eliminated in 18 to 24 hours—or less.

Some foods may have a wonderful taste,
But they produce lots of toxic waste
Uric acid in the bloodstream is carcinogenic
Roast beef may be tasty, but is flirting with cancer worth it?

Ayurvedic advice, a word to the wise:
Never eat to full stomach, whatever your size
Leave enough room so you can digest
Following proportions are deemed to be best:
With solid food fill half, with liquids, one quarter
This division is how the Vedas say we ought to
Handle your diet for health and well-being
Chew your food well, saliva you're needing

No teeth in the stomach, so don't gulp it down
Digestion starts in the mouth — and smile, don't frown!
Laughter is the best medicine, it's medically true
Have a sense of humor, whatever you do.

The human need for protein is highly overrated
You can get all you require in the foods that I've stated
Buy a cookbook, dare to try
Eating to live before you die.

A trio of friends I'd like you to meet:
Garlic, onions, and ginger will make your life sweet.
Onions purify blood and fight disease
Garlic makes you potent as semen increases
Ginger root strengthens nerve centers in the spine
Drinking ginger tea eases menstrual pain.

A dangerous spice I shall now introduce
Be very careful in its handling and use
When it's wet and it spills on your clothes
It's hard to wash out (believe me I know!)

What is the spice that does all this?
It's called "turmeric," put it on your shopping list.
Fantastically healing and tasty too
Makes bones and joints flexible—a tiny bit will do.
Golden milk you can make, the recipe's here
Serve it to all the folks you hold dear.

Yogi Tea, more than a beverage, a formula for health
Which, as you know, you can't buy with wealth
Each ingredient a purpose to serve
A scientific blend, a recipe to cure.
Help your digestion, prevent colds and flu
No medical claims (of course), but this is what the yogis do.

12
Creatures of Habit

*T*here is no doubt that we are all creatures of habit. A huge proportion of what we do, how we feel, speak, relate, is simply habit. A saint has saintly habits, a criminal has criminal habits. I don't want to use the word "sinner." Thinking of themselves as sinners has caused people too much damage already. I don't subscribe to the idea of sin, except as the Vedantists say, the sin of being ignorant of your divine nature.

Habits control us so strongly that it is said we can actually change our destiny by changing our habits. According to ancient yogic wisdom, there are six specific areas of habitual behavior to be changed:

way of walking	**way of dealing**
way of talking	**way of eating**
way of dressing	**way of worship**

Of course, the best way to break a habit is to replace it with a different one. This is one way yogis practice the concept of "resist not evil."

TWO KINDS OF HABITS[1]

"It has been seen in our entire concept of life, that we are 15% slaves to a routine, to habit. Man must have certain habits without which his life cannot go on. But he can attain liberation by changing the character of these minimum-required habits.

"There are two kinds of habits: promoting habits and demoting habits. Demoting habits make you unhappy physically, mentally, and spiritually. Promoting habits make you happy physically, mentally, and spiritually. In your life, if you have all the habits which are promoting habits, you will end up as a liberated, divine person. If you have demoting habits, you will always end up as a physical wreck, mentally insane, and/or spiritually defunct.

97

"Habit is a must of your personality and mind. For that period when you are acting under a demoting habit, you are totally in the negative personality. It is also a fact that if you get into any one negative habit, you will automatically attract its four sister habits, for they love to stay together. These five demoting habits of behavior and attitude are: greed, anger, lust, attachment, and negative ego. When one sister enters the house, she calls the others to join.

It takes 40 days to establish a habit, 90 days to confirm it, 120 days—everyone will know it!

"Each habit is supported on two tripods:
- Physical, Mental, and Spiritual,
- Past, Present, and Future.

"There are two guiding instincts in man. He is either improving his future or blocking his future improvement. If you are conscious of this, and have an honest and sincere urge to improve your future, you will always have promoting habits. Oh man, if you are to care not even for God, at least care for the future. When you care enough for your future to have promoting habits, you will become a liberated person.

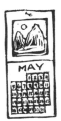

"A liberated person is always a happy person. He does not lack in any material comfort. He does not know any power on Earth which can insult him. He lives in grace in this world and when he leaves the body he is respected for generations to follow. Everyone can be like that.

"Yesterday's greatest sinner can be a saint this minute. The only thing required is a decision: 'Am I to guard my future and choose to be a liberated person, or am I to block my future and go by the material-physical aspect of the world?' ...Maintain a positive attitude with promoting habits for forty days, and you can change your destiny."

There is a fundamental meditation that works on changing habit patterns. It's called the **SA-TA-NA-MA** meditation. You'll find the original form that Yogi Bhajan first taught it in this book. Later he gave a beautiful visualization technique to practice with it. I've included that for you as an optional bonus-extra. I think you will enjoy it.

You will also find a breath meditation designed to help control addictive behavior (habits).

SUGGESTED PROMOTING HABIT

Do one special meditation every day for forty days. Keep a diary of your progress, and the changes you go through.

13
Drugs

"The Chinese took opium and lost their civilization. Indians took marijuana and lost their civilization. The Egyptians used peyote and other herbs and they lost their civilization. The Greeks and Romans lost their civilization with alcohol. The United States has them all."

—Yogi Bhajan

Why do people take drugs? To get out of facing reality. But drugs take you to non-reality. The use of drugs has become so widespread now, it's even considered "fashionable." Yet thousands of people continue to die from drugs and thousands of lives, careers, and marriages are destroyed by drug abuse. Babies are born already addicted because their mothers were users. The new "designer" drugs are even more lethal and dangerous than the drugs commonly used in the '60s. In 1994 a promising young actor, just twenty-two years old, River Phoenix, collapsed in front of a club in Beverly Hills and died shortly thereafter, another victim — of what? Drugs? Ignorance? Arrogance? ("It won't happen to me.") Social pressure?

When Yogi Bhajan arrived in Los Angeles in December of 1968, the "drug culture" was a way of life for almost an entire young generation. They had started taking drugs in order to find God. They had rejected society's material values and they wanted to experience spirit. Yes, they wanted to get "high," but for the majority it was a sincere spiritual quest, not just thrill-seeking.

Unfortunately, they didn't know the results of taking those drugs. They didn't know how much they would suffer from the side-effects. Out of twenty million young people, millions died, were permanently damaged, or went insane.

For those of you who were not there and do not remember the 60s (and for those of you who were there and do not remember the 60s), the following quote from Yogi Bhajan will illustrate the point:

"There is a possibility that some of you might feel, once in a while, to remember the '60s. Some of you are very innocent. You do not understand. I was addressing one situation today. At one time that person had taken so much drugs that the neurons in the brain were damaged. You have seven plates of neurons. If a plate is damaged because of acceleration and contraction, you can understand the subtle damage. It is just like a car which has a very weak battery. The caffeine, the stimulants, and all these things, at that moment may help you. But over a long time, they damage you."

When the Siri Singh Sahib, then known simply as "Yogiji," saw the condition the young people were in from having taken drugs, his compassion was aroused and impelled him to teach them Kundalini Yoga. He knew it was the fastest way to heal their bodies and minds, and give them the spiritual awakening they were seeking. He decided to teach Kundalini Yoga publicly, in spite of the fact that traditionally, because of the power it gives, it was forbidden to do so.

He understood their drive to use drugs was an attempt to change their consciousness, to fill an inner emptiness. They took drugs because they had not been taught any other way to take control of their inner lives. Drugs were a rejection of inner pain and stagnant mental states. But drugs did not provide a way to build any real basis for a new consciousness. He knew that Kundalini Yoga creates immediate, actual changes in consciousness. Although many drug users thought of Kundalini Yoga as another way to get "high," it is a way to becoming the higher self! It is getting out of pain, subconscious turmoil, and boredom. It does give you energy from within that cannot be given or created by any outside substance.

Yogi Bhajan knew that by doing Kundalini Yoga, the students would not only experience an even higher "high," but they would be repairing their nervous system and brain. He said it would take three years of doing Kundalini Yoga and eating a healthy diet to repair the damage that drugs had done. That was the beginning of the 3HO Drug Rehabilitation Program. We even stamped all of our 3HO outgoing mail with the slogan:

"Make this a drug-free nation.

Help the 3HO Foundation."

Yogi Bhajan never told students outright to stop taking drugs, but he pointed out the effects of taking them, and he gave simple things to do as an alternative:

When you feel the urge for some stimulant, take seven long deep breaths, holding each inhalation to the maximum. Or (if you're not out in public, that is), do Breath of Fire. It is the most powerful remedy!

"If you do a half-hour of Breath of Fire every day, there are a lot of troubles that you can keep miles away.[1]"

He let people discover for themselves they could get higher on Kundalini Yoga than on anything else. He pointed out that it's a permanent spiritual experience. There are no damaging side-effects. It's also legal and less expensive than drugs. Not only did every yoga class help heal past damage, but it gave an immediate "up" experience.

> **When you feel the urge for a stimulant take seven long deep breaths, holding each inhalation to the maximum. Or (if you're not out in public, that is), do Breath of Fire. It is the most powerful remedy!**

Armed with Yogi Bhajan's masterful technology, a special full-care, drugless 3HO Drug Rehabilitation facility in Tucson, Arizona, was begun. Staffed by qualified professionals, it evolved into "SuperHealth," a haven for anyone wanting to relax, rejuvenate, and regenerate. Using Kundalini Yoga as the main feature of the program, guests or clients were given massage, counseling, diet, and motivational techniques to improve the quality of their lives.

"Recreational drugs" is an oxymoron. Drugs neither create nor re-create, they destroy.

MARIJUANA

Not even marijuana is "safe." Marijuana attacks the nerve centers in the spine. Therefore, the entire nervous system, all 72,000 nerves in the body, are damaged. Another major effect of marijuana is damage to the memory function.

The two hemispheres of the brain expand and contract depending upon the activity of the nostrils. What happens when a person smokes "pot" is that whichever nostril is "open" expands the corresponding hemisphere of the brain. This creates the euphoric experience and the distortion of space perception and vision, "spaciness." The problem is that whenever the brain is affected by drugs, its usual control factor of the expansion and contraction is destroyed. From then onward, whether the person is smoking "grass" or not, that hemisphere can expand any time, any place. People get spaced out, forget what they are doing from one moment to the next. My observation was that marijuana made the most intelligent people incompetent and undependable. Marijuana stimulates the brain cells and it constricts the spinal fluid.

Yogi Bhajan pointed out to us that marijuana grows wild in India, but nobody bothers to smoke it anymore, because they know its disastrous effects.

SLEEPING PILLS

Thirty-five million people in this country cannot sleep at night. Many take sleeping pills. Sleeping pills make you neurotic, because they make the body sleep, but they do not let the subconscious sleep. Everything gets pushed into the unconscious. And when things get put into the unconscious, man is a living "crazy." He has absolutely no nervous control system. The parasympathetic doesn't even come through. And there's not yet a medicine which can cure this disease, because they do not deal with the root cause. They just cover the surface.

Yogiji taught us the yogic procedure for how to go to sleep at night without pills, sleep better and deeper, and wake up refreshed. You can read all about it in the chapter on *Sleep.*

CYCLES OF LIFE

Human beings have three distinct time periods, or cycles when major changes take place. These are in the realms of consciousness (seven years), intelligence (eleven years), and physical (eighteen years).

During the first eighteen years of life, the body is growing, so it seems as if we can get away with just about anything without noticing any ill effects. Kids can eat junk food, go without sleep, get no exercise, even smoke and drink, and still feel pretty good. From eighteen to thirty-six the body goes on reserve and so it still seems as if we can get away with unhealthy habits because the body is using its strong recuperative power to adjust and adapt. But after the age of thirty-six, look out! All the damage we have done, all the abuse and the neglect of the health of our physical body comes back to haunt us. We're no longer on reserve. The body starts to manifest the effects of all the past misuse and abuse. We get the aches and pains: bursitis, arthritis, and digestive problems that seem to come with age. It's not age folks, it's deficiency.

Fortunately, it's never too late to try to improve conditions. Even if you are over thirty-six, don't despair. By practicing Kundalini Yoga you have already begun to mend and repair, heal, and strengthen your body.

Kundalini Yoga is not necessarily "easy" —because you have to DO it, you don't just pop a pill in your mouth, or stick a needle in your arm. Two of Yogi Bhajan's earliest sayings are worth quoting here. They are true!

There's no freedom which is free.
There's no liberation without labor.

"I know you may have taken LSD, you may have taken PCP, but you can get rid of the after-effects of these drugs if you are honest with sadhana, (regular daily spiritual practice). This is how it works. These kinds of drugs, stimulants, uppers, downers (include sleeping pills in this category), no matter what they are, control the opening and closing capacity of the working of the brain's metabolism. It is permissible to take a drug only under dire medical emergency. Otherwise, in any normal functioning brain, when you take drugs, you make it function abnormally. A lot of people who stick to sadhana *(See chapter on Sadhana)* have been found to be totally clear of the effects and abnormalities created by the use of drugs. An abnormality includes any physical, mental, or spiritual abnormality. That is why sadhana has been designated and designed in three parts: one part relates to the physical, the second part relates to the mental, and the third part relates to the spiritual. We want to dispense this every morning with the idealistic thought that the person may gradually benefit from it.

"If you have to be addicted to something, be addicted to doing sadhana daily. Otherwise, addiction is not a source of freedom. And you are not free by taking drugs. The neurons of the brain will become feeble. Take the drugs. What's it to me? But it's you who will lose your nostril pituitary sensitivity. You can never smell the subtlety of life. You'll always be dragging your life."[2]

COCAINE

Cocaine gives a person a false sense of invincibility, and that, of course, is especially appealing to young people. I guess they don't believe all the statistics that demonstrate that cocaine is an addiction that is usually fatal. Or maybe they believe it but they think it can't happen to them. We all tend to think that disasters happen to "other people," not to us.

HABIT OR ADDICTION?

Behavior patterns are the result of the radiance of the psyche and frequency of the magnetic field in relationship to the universal psyche and magnetic force. When I first heard Yogi Bhajan explain this, I had to write it down and read it over and over to understand it. What is important to understand is that we all have habit patterns. We could not function without them. However, we often outgrow the patterns that we've created. We change, so we want to change our patterns. Or, we want to change because we know that by changing our habit patterns, we can change our lives!

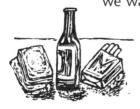

Whether it's overeating, taking drugs, smoking, drinking, or gambling, we can get into habits that can be very self-destructive. How to change these patterns? Increase your frequency. The tool for doing this is the mantra **SA TA NA MA** which is the nuclear form of the seed sound, **SAT NAM**. Mantra means mind projection. It is a technical device for regulating the mind. *(See chapter on Mantra.)* The **SA TA NA MA** meditation was introduced in the *Let's Talk About Food* chapter, and referred to again in *Creatures of Habit*. Here's more information about why these syllables are so effective.

Seed sounds or "Bij" mantras are sounds which totally rearrange the habit patterns of the subconscious mind. By vibrating the sound current of **SAT NAM** you activate that particular energy in the mind that erases and establishes habits. It represents the sound embodiment of Truth itself: **SAT** (truth) is the reality of what exists and **NAM** (name, identity) is the vibration which creates what it names. **SA TA NA MA** is the basic evolutionary force in the human psyche, and its effect is the same as splitting the atom.

SA is the infinite, the beginning. **TA** is life: from the infinite comes life and existence. **NA** is death: from life comes death or change. From death comes the Consciousness of the joy of the infinite, which leads back to life, **MA**, or rebirth.

Turn the page for a meditation for Breaking Addiction, using this "Bij" mantra...

"Difficult things take a long time;
The impossible takes a little longer."[3]

BREAKING ADDICTION
By Rearranging Your Subconscious Mind

In this meditation, the thumbs rest against the temples. The pressure exerted by the thumbs triggers a rhythmic reflex current directly underneath the stem of the pineal gland. It is imbalance in this obscure area that makes mental and physical addiction seemingly unbreakable.

Imbalance in the area below the pineal upsets the pulsating radiance that regulates the pituitary gland. Since the pituitary regulates the rest of the glandular system, the entire body and mind go out of balance when the pineal is dormant. This meditation corrects the problem. It is excellent for everyone, but particularly effective for rehabilitation efforts in drug dependence, mental illness, and phobic conditions.

Although this meditation will produce results within 5 to 7 minutes, work up to a maximum of 31 minutes a day. Human habit patterns are set or broken in forty-day cycles. More deeply ingrained patterns may take longer to correct.

Once the pineal gland has started secreting, it will give you radiance. It will free you from old patterns.

Sit in a comfortable pose. Straighten the spine and make sure the first six lower vertebrae are locked forward. Make fists of both hands and extend the thumbs out straight. Place the thumbs on the temples where there is a small indentation about an inch beyond the eyebrows. This is the lower anterior portion of the frontal bone above the temporal-sphenoidal suture.

Lock the back molars together and keep the lips closed. Vibrate the jaw muscles by alternating the pressure on the molars with the rhythm of **SA TA NA MA**. A muscle will move under the thumbs. Feel it massage the thumbs and apply a firm pressure with the hands.

Keep the eyes closed and look toward the brow point. Silently vibrate the syllables **SA TA NA MA** there. Continue 5 to 7 minutes, working up to 31 minutes over a period of daily practice sessions.

14
Sleep

"Sleep that knits up the ravell'd sleave of care."[1]

Have you ever had insomnia? Have you ever had to take sleeping pills? Do you sometimes wake up in the morning feeling as if you've been run over by a ten-ton truck, or stepped on by an elephant? Do you think you need more sleep? Do you wish you could get along on less sleep? This chapter is for you!

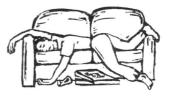

The purpose of sleep is to allow the body and the mind to rest, recuperate, regenerate — and do some self-healing. You should wake up rested, refreshed, and alert, ready to face the day. Do you?

FOUR STAGES OF SLEEP

There are several stages of sleep:

1. The first stage is the tossing and turning and worrying stage. It's a big waste of time and energy. It's not necessary to go through it at all, if you prepare yourself properly for sleep!

2. Next is usually a light dream, "reverie" stage (also not required), from which you go into an even more energy-draining stage:

3. Dream state. You may think you enjoy your dreams, but the fact is that whatever adventures you experience while you're dreaming take ten times more energy out of you than if the events actually happened while you were awake. No wonder you wake up exhausted. Especially if you're being chased by tigers, or attacked by monsters from outer space. We don't need to experience this state either. What we want to do, what we're aiming to reach, is:

4. The deep, dreamless sleep state. It is only in this fourth stage of sleep that we are actually rejuvenated, and our batteries get recharged.

Exploding the eight-hour myth.

HOW MUCH SLEEP DO I NEED?

Now that you're not going to waste precious time in the first three stages of sleep, you don't need eight hours of "sleep," honest!

Here's why: When your breath becomes erratic, when it is not slow and steady, it tears down your nervous system. After between four and a half to five and a half hours of sleep, your rate of breathing changes, so it's not a good idea to sleep any longer than that at one stretch. The deep sleep state actually only lasts a maximum of two and a half hours. The faster you can access the deep sleep stage, the less time you have to spend in the other stages. However, most of us take a little while to get into the deep sleep state and a little while to come out.

A healthy, full-grown adult living a reasonably healthy lifestyle really doesn't need to sleep more than five and a half hours! (It is said that those who have perfected their sleep skills can get all the benefits they need in only 31 minutes!)

Such great achievers as Madame Curie and Thomas Edison were known for their ability to take periodic "cat naps." They never slept for long hours at a time. One of the yogic powers much to be desired is the conquest of sleep! Being able to rejuvenate yourself in just a few minutes is a great asset in life. According to an article in the L.A. Times,[2] "President John F. Kennedy used to work in the Oval Office until 2 or 3 a.m. and then get up at 7:30 a.m., with daily one-hour naps. President Clinton tries to get by on five hours and a nap. Salvador Dali felt he only needed four hours of sleep a day. When overtired, he used to sit holding a spoon over a tin plate on the floor. When he fell asleep, he'd drop the spoon, waking himself up, claiming to be completely refreshed. Leonardo Da Vinci decided to sleep five minutes every four hours, a total of a half-hour each day. After five months he gave up—reporting that he felt all tingly around the head and was biting his tongue frequently—and went back to his regular four hours."

Well, obviously, Da Vinci went a bit overboard. However, we can learn how to relax so completely that just an eleven-minute nap can do wonders (in addition to a good yogic night's sleep, of course). In fact, taking two such eleven minute naps every day is highly recommended, especially for women.[3]

Unfortunately, many of us go to bed so loaded with anxiety that our minds keep going over and over the same problems and concerns, like a broken record. We even worry about whether we'll be able to go to sleep or not, and that keeps us awake. If we do fall asleep, it's a restless sleep.

It's a vicious circle: if our sleep is restless, then our rate of breathing becomes erratic. If the breath is erratic, the mind is disturbed. If we are mentally disturbed in sleep, the deep sleep stage may never be reached. Result: We wake up more tired than when we went to bed.

EAST-WEST IS BEST

For maximum efficiency and benefit from sleep, place your bed so that it is positioned east/west. Yes, you want to sleep in a line that cuts across the earth's magnetic field.

Just as the needle of a compass is always pulled toward the north, your personal energy will get swallowed up by the pull of the earth's magnetic field unless you sleep with your electromagnetic field at right angles to it. Positioning your bed north/south could be the reason you wake up tired and grouchy in the morning.

Your entire nervous system is affected by the direction in which you sleep. It doesn't matter which end your head is at, the important thing is to have the lines of force in your body going east-west. East-West is Best!

"Two worst enemies of your spine are automobiles and SOFT BEDS." We all need to walk more and drive less.

BE KIND TO YOUR SPINE

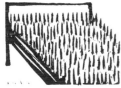

A soft bed may feel cozy, but to support your spine properly, and get the best night's sleep, you need a very firm surface to sleep on. This isn't meant to torture you. It's not necessary (or even desirable) to sleep on a bed of nails. But if you want to give maximum relaxation to your entire nervous system, you have to give maximum support to your spinal column. All 72,000 nerves in your body are connected to those twenty-six vertebrae in your spine.

So, "Good-bye waterbed," "So long, thick feather mattress!"

109

Get the firmest mattress you can find. Or try a three-inch futon or foam pad. You need to get rid of soft, non-supporting beds in order to experience the rest and relaxation you need and deserve. Many people who can afford every luxury still choose to sleep with only a Persian rug and a sheepskin for padding on a carpeted floor!

Okay, now you know how to get your bed ready. There's more to do before you get into it.

SIX STEPS TO PREP FOR SLEEP

First, make sure you've done some good strenuous exercise during the day, so that your physical body is ready and eager to rest. Everybody needs to exercise enough to sweat every day. A walk before bedtime is wonderful.

Second, don't eat a heavy meal just before bedtime. If your stomach is full, the digestive process will demand a lot of activity, just when all systems should be slowing down for sleep.

Third, brush your teeth to get rid of bacteria-forming food particles. Brush the root of the tongue also, to clear out pockets of mucous at the back of the throat.

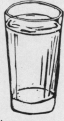

Fourth, don't go to bed thirsty. Drink at least one or two glasses of water before you go to sleep, even if you have to get up during the night to go to the bathroom. That is better than going to sleep thirsty. When the body is dehydrated, it demands water. That demand will disturb the mind, preventing proper rest and can even cause bad dreams. Children, who have pretty good instincts (until we stifle them), usually ask for a glass of water before bedtime. Give it to them.

Fifth, run some cold water over your feet, or soak them in cold water. Yes, COLD water! Then dry them vigorously with a towel. This will stimulate the 72,000 nerve endings in the sole of each foot and help get your nervous system ready for deep relaxation and sleep. To make this even more effective, you're going to massage your feet as soon as you get into bed. Or, better yet (and this is the ultimate luxury), get someone to give you a foot massage! But wait, don't lie down yet, there are still a few more preliminary steps.

Sixth, exercise. Having made all these preparations, brushed your teeth, had a glass of water, and washed your feet, it's very useful to do a few Kundalini Yoga exercises.

Other ways to set yourself for successful sleep are to:
- Read something inspirational
- Say your prayers
- Meditate
- Turn on your auto-reverse tape recorder and play some beautiful meditative music while you sleep. Subliminal tapes do work.
- Now you're ready for a big treat. It's your foot massage!

If you don't have anyone handy to give you a foot massage, you can do it yourself. *(Complete instructions in the Things To Do section.)* By the way, if you want your husband, wife, sweetheart, child, parent, or sibling to totally adore you, give them a foot massage! It is the kindest, most soothing, comforting act of healing.

There's one more very important thing to do before you go to sleep:

To be sane, two things you need to do every day: SWEAT & LAUGH!

(Maybe you can laugh while you're out walking!)

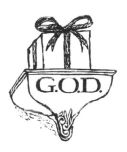

Before you go to sleep, take all your worries, concerns, ideas, and problems, wrap them up in a package and put them on a shelf in your mind labeled, "G - O - D." Leave them there. You'll be amazed at how many are gone, solved, and improved by the time you wake up. The whole package may have vanished!

Don't forget to set your mental timer to wake you up in the morning Yes, your subconscious mind has a great sense of time. It will respond to your directive. Just before you go to sleep, tell yourself what time you're going to wake up. At first you'll probably also want to use an alarm clock, just for insurance. You'll be surprised how quickly you can develop your own internal wake-up system. This ability will come in handy when you want to practice "How to Wake Up in the Morning" the yogic way.

In the Beginners Kundalini Yoga Series, I teach a special breath meditation to practice at bedtime. It's in the *Things To Do* section, along with some exercises that work well at bedtime.

Now you're ready for the yogic secret to deep sleep:

FOUR SIMPLE STEPS
TO DEEP, DREAMLESS SLEEP

Even if you haven't followed all the preliminary steps to the letter (but you're wise if you do!), you can still try this routine when you finally do lie down:

1. Lie on your stomach and turn your head so that your right cheek is on the pillow (or the bed as you prefer). This will automatically free up your left nostril to bring in the cooling, soothing, calming energy.

2. Start long deep breathing, inhaling maximum, exhaling maximum. Of course, you are ONLY breathing through your nose, keeping your mouth closed. Breathe consciously. Concentrate on making each breath as long and deep as you can. Think the sound SAT as you inhale, and NAM as you exhale.

3. After a few long deep breaths, use your arm or hand to completely block your right nostril. Continue long deep breathing only through the left nostril.

4. When you feel yourself reaching a slight stage of drowsiness, which usually takes about ten complete breaths, turn over onto your back or your side as you wish, depending upon how you are most comfortable. Continue long deep breathing until you are fast asleep! By the way, it is better for your heart and your digestion to sleep on the right side than the left. Plus, of course, it keeps your left nostril open.

As soon as the breath becomes regular and slow, you will go quickly through the preliminary stages of sleep and almost immediately reach the deep dreamless sleep state, avoiding the energy draining dream stage altogether. Plus you'll be able to come back out of deep sleep more easily and gracefully when it's time to wake up.

TECHNICAL STUFF

In case you're interested, here's a more scientific explanation of the yogic terms for some stages of sleep as described by MSS Gurucharan Singh Khalsa, Ph.D., who knows all the technical terms. I just know what works!

Awake is normal awareness of earth and defining the self by circumstances and outer objects.

Jugarat (or however it is spelled) is the self with the sense of the inner world: dreams, images, psychic impressions, the subconscious storages of self.

Soopan is heavy dream stage. (Very exhausting!)

Skoopat, or dreamless, is beyond the pull of the five elements and into the sense of merged spirit where identity is not based on the world.

Turiya is awakened sleep. Awake as Infinite Spirit and aware of the other realms of self. That is why Yogi Bhajan says he knows nothing about dreams. "I never had one." He has a state of Turiya in which Reality of Self is always present. The subconscious absorption into dreams and symbols is not needed. A symbol experienced in Turiya is a vision or an intuition.

$\mathcal{S}$LEEPY TIME SONG

Shakespeare said t'was "Sleep that knits up the ravell'd sleave of care—"
I guess he never had insomnia, nor dreamed he was chased by a bear

Sweet dreams are not so sweet at all
They take ten times the energy to run or fall
T'would take if t'were happening awake
So, yogis say, "avoid dreaming, for heaven's sake!"

Drink some water at bedtime we recommend
Give your stomach a rest — it will be your friend

Put your troubles on a shelf before you retire
Mark it "G-O-D" and see what transpires
In the morning they may be gone forever
Meanwhile, forget them overnight - aren't you clever?

Breathing slower and slower, your mind slows down too
Left nostril engaged, sweet Morpheus woo
Deeper and deeper you drift away
To awake refreshed to a brand new day

Prepare your body, instruct your mind
Sleeping becomes a pleasure you'll find!

A foot massage is a bonus delight
Sets your nerves at peace for the night
(Wash feet first in cold water - feels great)
Play your auto-reverse with an inspiring tape

Firm mattress placed east and west
(Yogis concur, this is the best)
Do some exercise — you can't go wrong
And this is the end of my Sleepytime song!

15
How to Get Up in the Morning

"When you wake, tell yourself you are bountiful, blissful, and beautiful:

Bountiful—when you know your soul

Blissful—neither pain nor pleasure affects you

Beautiful—in adversity you speak the language of prosperity

Do you think to give thanks for your arms and your legs? Your eyes and ears? In those moments as you come out of the sleep state, acknowledge how wonderful is this vehicle the Creator manufactured for you to use during your visit to planet Earth."

—Yogi Bhajan

THE WAY THE YOGIS DO IT...

You can, of course, set an alarm, have a wake-up service phone you, or ask someone to call you. But ideally (if you're smart), you will have consciously set your inner alarm the night before by telling your sub-conscious what time you want to get up. The subconscious mind has a very accurate sense of time and will be happy to serve you!

Always come out of sleep slowly and gradually. No sudden moves! Be kind to your nervous system.

If you leap out of bed when the alarm rings, that abrupt transition from sleep to waking is a shock that damages your nervous system. Instead of the jumping-jack scenario, when it's time to wake up, try this:

KEEP YOUR EYES CLOSED

Inhale very deeply and stretch your arms way up and back over your head. Take a few long deep breaths, s-t-r-r-r-e-t-c-h-i-n-g your spine, and then do a:

CAT STRETCH

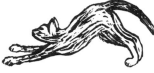

Bend one knee up to your chest and swing it across the front of your body to touch the bed on the opposite side; then do the same thing with the other knee. Twist and turn and bend to the maximum. This is good for your circulation and for the nervous system. You are letting the electromagnetic field balance itself.

Stretching first thing in the morning is a major factor in helping you go through the day balanced and calm. Be sure to do it.

THE EYES HAVE IT !

You've done all the stretching with your eyes closed. Now, lying flat on your back, put the palms of your hands tightly over your closed eyes. Then, but not until then, open your eyes, look directly into the palms of your hands. Slowly — very slowly, continue to gaze at your palms (reading your fortune?) as you lift your hands straight up to about eighteen inches above your face. This gives your optic nerve a chance to adjust gradually to the light and distance, and helps to keep your eyesight strong. Protect your eyesight, always avoid any sudden shock of light.

WAKE UP YOUR FACE

From the eighteen-inch height, bring your fingertips down to the center of your forehead, and with a circular motion, massage your forehead from the center out to the temples and down both sides of the face to the tip of your chin. (There are special pressure points on either side of the chin, which are lunar centers.) Now massage your nose and your ears, squeeze your nostrils and your ear lobes briefly to get the circulation going. Take a few more long deep breaths to open up your lungs and get ready for:

STRETCH POSE

Lying on your back, legs straight, bring your heels together and lift your head and your heels about six inches off the bed (twelve inches, maximum), balancing on your buttocks, while keeping your eyes open and focusing steadily on your big toes (or the blankets covering the toes!). Hold the position for one minute with Breath of Fire. Arms are held straight at your sides, palms facing your thighs, but not touching. (Sort of like a sentry at Buckingham Palace, except that you can smile.) If your eyes water, that's OK, it's good lubrication for them. If your body shakes, that's okay. It indicates the nervous system is adjust-

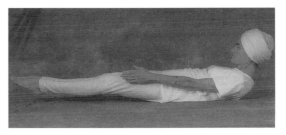

ing. If you can't maintain stretch pose for the full minute, do it in segments, even if it's only ten seconds at a time. Just do the best you can, and keep trying! It's time well spent because:

Stretch pose adjusts your navel point. Since the navel is the focal point for all 72,000 nerves in the body, stretch pose is a tune-up for your whole nervous system as well as your digestive system. It also strengthens your reproductive organs and glands (the seat of your creativity and productivity).

NOSE TO KNEES

After one minute of stretch pose, relax for about 15 seconds and then bend your knees to your chest, hold them tight against your body, lift your head and put your nose right in between your knees. In this position do Breath of Fire for 30 seconds to one minute, pumping your navel. This stimulates the apana (outgoing life breath) and helps your elimination. Just as prana is not breath itself, but carried on the incoming life breath, apana is the eliminating force of the body, carried on the outgoing, or eliminating breath. It is the cleansing breath of life that gets rid of the toxins. Add to the benefit of this exercise by mentally repeating the mantra **WAHE GURU** or **SAT NAM** over and over in your mind, synchronized with the breath. Hear it loud and clear as you inhale and exhale. Then inhale deeply, exhale, and relax the breath as you...

HAVE A HEART!

Keeping your knees tightly clasped to your chest, turn briefly onto your right side and rest for a minute or two. This posture strengthens the heart.

**Warning: this posture may be dangerous—
you're liable to fall back to sleep and be late for work.**

TAKE A WALK

Now you're ready to get out of bed and walk to the bathroom. Don't put on your slippers yet. It's better to go barefoot, so that your body can discharge any excess electromagnetic energy you've accumulated overnight. The first stretching you did in bed was to break through the "cocoon" of your individual electromagnetic field and reestablish contact with earth. Touching the walls and touching the faucets with both hands will help continue the process of "grounding yourself" for the day ahead.

BATHROOM ALERT

As we explain in the chapter called, "Let's Talk About Food," when you go to the toilet first thing in the morning, you can verify how well you are digesting your food by looking to see if your stool floats. If it does, it means your body has gotten the benefit of all the food value in whatever you ate, and it is just eliminating what it could not use to build blood, bone, and tissue. If your stool sinks, then something is wrong, either with your diet or with your digestive system, and probably both. And, you can tell by the color of your urine how your kidneys are doing. The color should not be darker than gold.

BRUSH YOUR TONGUE

Not just to whiten and brighten your teeth, but for the sake of your health, here is a yogic recipe for oral hygiene: Take two parts powdered potassium alum[1] mixed with one part of common household salt and use it like tooth powder to brush your teeth. More importantly, brush the root of your tongue. Why?

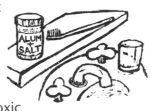

During the night, your mouth turns into an incubator, warm, moist, and cozy. In that environment, bacteria have an orgy and they multiply like crazy. Unless you get rid of that toxic accumulation, you will swallow it with the first sip of liquid. So, to avoid poisoning yourself, use your toothbrush and reach way back to the root of your tongue until you gag and cough up that disease-producing mucous. The two little glands back there called "monkey glands" need to be cleaned out.

Another benefit is that as you gag, it makes your eyes water. Ancient yogis called that "cataract" water, and said that it helps preserve the eyesight. So, a word to the wise: use this astringent combination of alum and salt every morning. I keep the mixture in a clean, dry, empty mustard jar. I pour a little, about the size of a quarter, in the palm of one hand, wet my toothbrush and dip it in. You can finish with your favorite toothpaste on your teeth, if you wish. I do.

OIL AND WATER, THE BEST MIXTURE

Next on the morning agenda is the biggest challenge of the day, the ever popular 3HO trademark, the COLD SHOWER! But first, before you get under

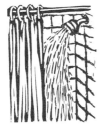

the shower, yes, before you get wet, massage your body all over with a little oil. Oil is more easily absorbed by the skin when it is mixed with water—and you won't be greasy afterwards. Almond oil is highly recommended since the almond contains so many minerals, and it nourishes the body through the pores of your skin. Go for it! When the cold water hits the surface of your skin (which has four layers) all the blood from way deep inside your body rushes to the surface in self-defense, vastly improving your circulation on the spot. This is called hydrotherapy. It strengthens your entire nervous system. People pay huge sums of money for what is now called

"Hydrothermal therapy," when in reality all you need is your own two hands, cold water, and courage.

An added benefit is that you will probably become very holy the moment the cold water hits your body, because it is very likely you will shout, "Oh my God!" You might try exclaiming, "*Wahe Guru*" ("Wow, God is Great!") or "*Ang Sang Wahe Guru*" ("God lives in every limb of my being.") Remembering God is always a blessing.

Go in and out of the water four times, constantly massaging your body until the water no longer feels cold. Be sure to get the arm-pits (major nerve centers) and the insides of the thighs. You can even stand on one foot and massage the top of it with the other foot, but don't slip or trip! Women, be sure to massage your breasts.

Then, your first victory of the day achieved, dry off briskly with a rough towel till the body really shines; put on loose, comfortable exercise clothing, and you're ready to do your sadhana, your personal daily spiritual practice. *(See Sadhana: Your Spiritual Bank Account.)* God bless you, you're bound to have a wonderful day!

"It's not the life that matters, it's the courage you bring to it." [2]

If you really love hot showers, wonderful. Take them at night, or sometime when you can wrap up afterwards in lots of blankets and sweat for at least an hour or two. But in the morning, cold water is your best friend. The morning shower is for your circulation, and stimulation of your nervous and glandular systems.

16
Sadhana: Your Spiritual Bank Account

Envy of the Angels
(Angels Can't Do Sadhana)

*I*t has been said that even the angels envy us because it is only when a being has evolved into the human form (after 8.4 million lifetimes in other forms), that he/she can be liberated from the cycle of birth and death. No other life form has this opportunity. Not even the angels.

To experience liberation we have to expand our awareness beyond the limitations of our individual consciousness. Only then can we merge into the vastness of the Universal Self, which is our true identity. That expansion takes courage and consistent effort. It takes work.

"THERE IS NO LIBERATION WITHOUT LABOR[1]"

The main work toward liberation is called sadhana. Sadhana is the base, the foundation of all spiritual endeavor. Sadhana is your personal, individual spiritual effort. It is the main tool you use to work on yourself to achieve the purpose of life. It can be done alone or with a group. Sadhana is whatever you do consistently to clear your own consciousness so you can relate to the infinity within you. To cover all your bases, it will include exercise, meditation, and prayer.

Before you face the world each day, before you go into your kitchen to fix breakfast, before you ride your bike to school, jog to your office, or get in your car to fight the battle of the freeways: do yourself a favor and tune up your nervous system and attune yourself to your highest inner self.

121

The power of your sadhana is enhanced by doing it with other people. To go from individual to universal consciousness, we have to go through group consciousness. Group sadhana develops group consciousness. You will find that communication and dealings with the people who do sadhana with you is much easier than with other people, because you have created an harmonious inner avenue of communication.

Have you hugged your soul today?

AMBROSIAL HOURS — RIGHT TIME / RIGHT PLACE

There are certain times of the day that are best suited for meditation: the ideal time slot is four o'clock to seven o'clock in the morning. Then, to make a positive transition from day to night-time, four to seven in the evening,

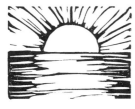

During what are called the "ambrosial hours" (the two and a half hours just before sunrise), when the sun is at a sixty-degree angle to the earth, the energy you put into your sadhana gets maximum results. Your world is quieter. It's easier to meditate and concentrate before the hustle and bustle of the day begins. This is the time we need to be awake to receive that first solar energy of the day. "Any fool can sleep, but wise is that one who rises before the sun."[2]

ARE YOU THINKING, "I CAN'T GET UP THAT EARLY!"?

If you absolutely cannot get up early in the morning to do sadhana, then do it some other time! Doing sadhana at any time of the day or night, will benefit you. However, it is a fact that the optimum time is during the ambrosial hours. As Yogi Bhajan says, "If you can't have the best, make the best of what you have." If you can't do sadhana for two and a half hours, do it for an hour; if you can't do it for an hour, do it for thirty-one minutes, or eleven minutes. If you don't want to do the sadhana outlined in this book, do some other sadhana, but for God's sake— (and your sake) —do something!

ONE HOLY MAN'S SPECIAL SADHANA

Once there was a very holy man who lived in a cave high in the mountains of the Himalayas. He practiced austerities and penances for many years. Every morning he would appear at the cave entrance just before sunrise, and stand waiting for the first rays of dawn to appear over the horizon, illuminating a spectacular panorama of hundreds and hundreds of miles of lush green forest. He could look down and see the mirrored reflection of his own snowcapped mountain shimmering in the crystal clear river sparkling miles below. Overwhelmed with the beauty of God's creation, he never tired of the exquisite sight. Awestruck at the wonder of God's creation that greeted his eyes each dawn, he watched the sun rise, clapped his hands in glee and shouted at the top of his lungs, "Well done, God, well done!" This was his way of giving thanks to his Creator. This was his sadhana.

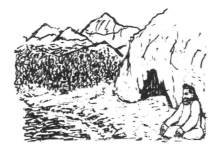

SUGGESTIONS: HOW TO DO MORNING SADHANA

PREPARATION

Morning sadhana really starts the night before. It starts with how you go to sleep at night, so you can wake up early in the morning the yogic way. One of the most essential steps in that preparation for morning sadhana is a cold shower. Yes, cold. People pay thousands of dollars for hydrothermal therapy, but you can achieve the same results for only a few cents a day in your own cold shower. I can't repeat often enough how valuable it is to take that cold shower. That's where you can open up your capillaries, increase your circulation, wake up and strengthen your entire nervous system in about five minutes. All you have to do is massage your body vigorously under cold water first thing in the morning until the water doesn't feel cold. After this "tune-up" you're ready to tune-in for your morning sadhana. I'm going to describe in detail the sadhana prescribed by Yogi Bhajan, and practiced by thousands of 3HO students throughout the world. Please join us!

LOCATION

It's best to do sadhana in the same place every day. Ideally, you will find a 3HO Yoga Center or Ashram, and participate in the group sadhana there. Everyone benefits from the combined energy. You can, of course, do your sad-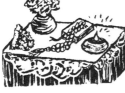hana at home. Just select a clean, quiet spot where you will not be disturbed. You may want to set up an altar of some kind with pictures, flowers, statues, whatever sets a mood of reverence for you. This altar becomes a focal point for your meditative energy.

After you tune in by chanting **ONG NAMO GURU DEV NAMO** (at least three times), do a set of Kundalini Yoga exercises (remember to include the relaxations), then you're ready to begin chanting.

MORNING MANTRAS

Sit in Easy Pose, on either wool or cotton padding of some sort. Some people use sheepskins, others prefer a folded blanket. Your foundation should be solid so you can sit still. You can chant sitting in a chair or even lying in bed if your physical condition requires it. Be sure to keep your spine as straight as you can.

The words for all seven of the morning sadhana mantras are at the end of this chapter. The sequence begins with seven minutes of chanting Long Ek Ong Kar's. This mantra opens all the chakras. *(See the Things To Do section for specific directions for chanting it.)* All of the other mantras for the morning may be chanted to your choice of melodies, with or without musical accompaniment. There are several audio tapes[3] available with different musical versions of all the "Aquarian Sadhana" mantras. Try them until you find one that suits you. Or, you can create your own melodies. But be sure to keep the same comparative length of syllables and maintain the same rhythm as they would be spoken if you were simply reciting them in a monotone, without any music. This attention to rhythm preserves the "Naad," which is the inner sound, the power, of the syllables. This is very important. Not every tape that has been produced is flawless in this regard, but as the scriptures say, "*Mantram Siddyam, Siddhyam Parameshwaram.*" He who masters mantra, masters God Himself. Perfection can't be expected to be easily achieved. You will have to be the best judge of which morning sadhana tape works best for you. One of the many advantages to group sadhana is that you can just surrender to the process, as someone else leads the exercises and the chanting. (Or, you can lead it and do it "your way!")

THE AGONY AND THE ECSTASY

I would like to say that morning sadhana will give you a blissful experience. I can't honestly promise you that. The fact is, sometimes it can be downright miserable. It is a cleansing process. Garbage accumulated from many lifetimes gets stirred up and comes floating to the surface. You may find yourself observing some very unpleasant, ugly thoughts while you're meditating or chanting. Garbage consists of such attitudes and feelings as anger,

125

resentment, fear, frustration, self-pity, depression, insecurity. The important thing is, keep on chanting! The mantras are doing their job. You're cleaning up and getting rid of the negativity that has been covering up the divine light inside you.

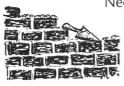

Negative vibrations create blocks of negativity. These blocks pile up forming walls of negativity, walls that separate us from experiencing the God inside us. It is this sense of separation that makes us unhappy. By continuing to chant, you're replacing negative vibrations with positive ones, and the walls come tumbling down!

If we don't clean up the subconscious on a regular basis, negativity continues to accumulate. When it reaches a saturation point, it spills over into the unconscious mind and then it's really hard to get rid of it.

To be truly liberated and in control of our minds and our lives, we can't be pushed and pulled around by irrational compulsions from the sub-conscious.

Praying is talking to God,meditating is letting God talk to you.

Did you ever do something you really didn't want to do? Or do something you now wish you hadn't done? Well, the desires and the compulsions to action or lack of action, caused by fear, come mostly from the sub-conscious. If we don't get rid of what's buried there, we can be in real trouble!

When you finish chanting for an hour—and even during that hour—remember to give thanks to your Creator. This is an excellent time to pray.

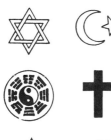

You have worked on your physical body with Kundalini Yoga exercises. You have worked on your mind, cleaning out the subconscious through chanting mantras, now it's time to refresh your spirit and integrate all parts of your being by offering yourself and dedicating your actions for the day to the One Creator who makes it possible for you to experience His marvelous creation. It's time for worship, however you choose.

It can be at your own altar, at your temple, church, or synagogue. We who are Sikhs go to the Gurdwara (literally, the "gate of the Guru") which is our temple. "Sikh" simply means student.

Everyone is welcome in any Sikh place of worship. People of all beliefs, castes, colors, genders, and ages are welcome. We bow when we first enter the Gurdwara. This is not only good for the circulation, but it allows us to express our intention to offer our lives in service to God and acknowledge that we

> **"God repects me when I work, but He loves me when I sing."**
> —Sufi Saying

belong to the Guru. We remind ourselves to "give our heads" to the Guru, offering our problems and worries to the Guru. Then we sing, offer a traditional prayer, listen to an excerpt from the Siri Guru Granth Sahib, to give us inspiration and guidance for the day. The Siri Guru Granth Sahib is a volume of sacred writings compiled from the words of Sikh Gurus as well as enlightened Hindu, Muslim, and Sufi saints all of whom experienced the highest state of Yoga. These words are, in effect, Words of God, and by reciting them and listening to them, we raise our consciousness. It is the Living Guru of the Sikhs. We then share some Gurprashad, a traditional sweet, made of whole wheat flour, honey, and clarified butter (literally: a "gift" of the Guru). Tasting this sweet mixture reminds us that everything we receive is sweet because everything comes from God. Then, as Sikhs, we are supposed to "go to work and earn righteously" so that we can have abundance to share with others.

The first Sikh Guru was Guru Nanak, who taught that God lives and breathes in everyone (sound familiar?) and that people should not fight about how to worship that One God. Therefore, Sikhs do not try to convert others to become Sikhs, and are committed to respecting—and even defending—the rights of others to worship however they choose.

HAVE A GOOD DAY

Having done sadhana, you have cleared your mind and consciously prepared yourself to go forth and be successful in handling whatever the day may bring. You consciously strive to hold on to the remembrance and the awareness of SAT NAM with every breath. Wherever you go, whatever you do, remember SAT NAM lives and breathes in you! (*Remember in the chapter on Breath of Life we said, "catch yourself breathing!"*)

127

$\mathcal{S}$ A D H A N A

Kundalini Yoga, meditation, and prayer
"Morning Sadhana," your soul wants to be there.
Be kind to your soul in the ambrosial hours
Get rid of impediments and experience your power.
You're already divine, a Spirit Being of Light
Clear away the debris so you can shine bright!

My mind can be a wonderful friend, and I truly love it dearly
But it doesn't always help me out, when I really need to think clearly.
Bombarded all day with sounds and sights
Cluttered with fantasies and dreams by night

Subconscious is constantly programmed subliminally
And the stuff we accumulate loads us down criminally
"Garbage in: garbage out," computer programmer knows
Subconscious garbage causes most of our woes

To clean it out, erase those files
It only takes a little while
Do sadhana each morning to get a fresh start
Raise your consciousness and open your heart

Series of mantras, one hour of chanting
Re-record on the disc of the mind
Sharpen your wits and hone your skills
These are just a few of the benefits you'll find

Sacred vibrations in scientific combination
Stimulate hypothalamus, change brain cells permutation

Chant God's Name before break of day
Sorrow and tension melt away
The process of cleansing I must admit,
Brings negativity to the surface - that's part of it
But unless it's removed, brought out to the light
It festers and multiplies — and that's not right!

Excess subconscious garbage not removed, overflows
Into your unconscious, that dark, murky, bottomless pit below.
Clean your mental house daily
It really is a must
Even if it does kick up a lot of dust

Any fool can sleep late and miss sun's first rays
But blessed be the soul who wakes to the day!
Two and a half hours before the sun rises
Best time for sadhana—practiced by the wisest.

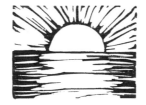

SPIRITUAL BANK ACCOUNT

Morning sadhana is the best investment in the world. It is like putting money in your spiritual bank account. It will always earn at least ten percent interest. For every hour of morning sadhana, you get ten hours of guidance and clarity! Therefore, the ideal sadhana lasts two and a half hours.

You can be sure when you're doing sadhana in the ambrosial hours that you're in the right place at the right time doing the right thing. What a great feeling of self-esteem and self-assurance, to start each day with that confidence! If you really want to "HAVE A GOOD DAY," sadhana is the way to begin it.

17
Woman is Spelled Double-You-O-Man

This chapter is written primarily for women,
but I think men will find it worth reading.
Shocking perhaps, but worth reading!

Our premise in this book is that everyone has the right to be healthy, happy, and holy. As women, there is a lot we can do to make this possible. Obviously something has to change. Any change starts with a change of attitude, a different idea, or concept. So I invite you to open your mind to a different way of viewing our lives, identity, and purpose as women. You may find some of the things you are about to read upsetting, but twenty-seven years of living, counseling, and observing the results of these ideas have convinced me of their practicality!

Yogi Bhajan pulls no punches. He strips away fantasy and teaches reality. This is not always a popular thing to do. He offers enlightened and universal knowledge of the true nature and characteristics of each gender. He has gone into great detail in hundreds of lectures and classes, explaining how men and women are different. Men may be "from Mars" and women may be "from Venus," but we're all here on Earth now, and we need to learn how to enjoy being here together.

It's obvious that the current belief system of the "equality" of men and women has not brought us happiness and fulfillment. Discontent, depression, and frustration are common. The divorce rate continues to grow and the fabric of society is torn by bitterness and resentment on both sides of the gender line. Though important, equal pay for equal jobs does not deal with the fundamental issue of our unique strengths and purpose as women and our impact on society.

"I believe that so long as those born of woman do not respect woman, there shall be no peace on Earth." —Yogi Bhajan

"You must win freedom and your right to be recognized as human. You cannot be paid less than a man, you can not be denied opportunities because you happen to be a woman. I am not asking you to become total tomboys, but I am telling you that the grace of woman demands to be treated nicely. She is the better half. If somebody opens the door for her it is no tragedy. It is a male courtesy to his own grace...I am not asking you to become feminists, but to be very graceful, absolute women."[1]

Adi Shakti Symbol

EVERY WOMAN IS A SHAKTI:
GOD'S POWER IN MANIFESTATION

Probably the most striking thing about Yogi Bhajan's attitude toward women is the place of respect and reverence he says is our God given right, and his insistence upon the nobility and invincibility of woman when she claims her rightful power and majesty as "Shakti."

The word Shakti means the feminine aspect of God, the Power through which "He" created the creation. Adi Shakti is the Primal Power.

THE POWER OF WOMEN

Men may not like to believe this, but women are actually sixteen times more powerful than men. Perhaps not in muscular strength, but a woman has sixteen times the emotional impact, sixteen times the intuitive awareness, and sixteen times the protective sense. She's the creature who endures childbirth. She's the one capable of turning her blood to milk to feed her child.

"God has given you sixteen times more courage and more comprehensive biological physical strength than a man. Have pity on this guy! He doesn't have all your biochemical action, doesn't have the mental lunar reflection, doesn't have the sophistication and softness and doesn't have the nervous system to deal with it, and he's still alive![2]"

Is it any wonder that a woman's influence and effect on a man can be enormous? Women throughout the ages have inspired men to greatness, or led them to their doom. What we say to a man can either elevate, inspire, and encourage him, or emasculate, antagonize, and sometimes destroy him. But, what about the exploitation of women? Yes, it is true, woman has been put-down, misused, abused, and brutally mistreated. But, this does not have to continue. When we acknowledge and accept our power as women, we can claim our rightful status of dignity, grace, and respect in society.

History shows that any society or civilization in which woman is not respected has ultimately been destroyed.

FROM A CHICK TO AN EAGLE: THE INVINCIBLE WOMAN

Recognizing the need to educate women about women, Yogi Bhajan created a special summer intensive training program for women. The first Khalsa Women's Training Camp, KWTC, (Khalsa means "pure one") was held in 1976, on land bought by Yogi Bhajan in Espanola, New Mexico. Camp ran for eight weeks, and the women ran, too! Everything from martial arts and marching, to music and meditation was taught. Yogi Bhajan personally lectured and led Kundalini Yoga classes every day. He was determined to elevate and transform woman in this country from a "chick" to an eagle! He emphasized the nobility of woman.

He taught special meditations for women, shared ancient secrets on health and diet for women. He lectured on virtually every aspect of a woman's life including love, romance (versus reality), marriage, and childraising, always building our self-esteem and reminding us of the divine nature of Woman. He told us, "You are the Grace of God."

Espanola still hosts KWTC each summer for several weeks, and women can even come for just a weekend of rejuvenation, inspiration, and education.

133

WHAT DOES A MAN KNOW ABOUT WOMEN?

Sometimes newcomers to camp wonder how a man can know so much about women.

For one thing, during his childhood in India, young Harbhajan Singh Puri had the unique experience of attending an all girls Catholic school. It was the only school available in the area where his family lived. So, Yogi Bhajan learned early in life to deal with many women. He tells stories of the hard time he gave the nuns with his constant questions: unnerving and to the point!

Yogi Bhajan's mother was a very powerful, righteous woman whose training had an impact on him which he has never forgotten. He cherishes her memory to this very day. He has never forgotten the values she taught him. But his understanding of women goes far beyond any male perspective.

As a Master, as a Yogi, Yogi Bhajan always sees women—and men—from a cosmic viewpoint. He never forgets that we are primarily souls, paying our karma and learning our lessons in these two different forms.

SUN and MOON

Cosmically speaking, the male carries the energy and the radiance of the sun, the female represents the moon, the lunar energy. She waxes and wanes. He does not. The sun is stationary, shining, and warm in spite of the clouds. The moon is bright, beautiful, and reflecting. Take these two elements and you can understand the character of man and woman. She shines her brightest reflecting the light of the sun. Reflect your man and you've got him. And if he's warm and shining, firm, stationary and stable, he wins her heart. Does that mean woman does not have her own identity? No, simply they are different. Without the moon to nourish and sustain, whatever grows from the solar energy will not last. Male and female are meant to complement and supplement each other. He is the seeder, she is the nourisher and sustainer. She is meant to contain the male, just as the word female contains the male, and the word woman contains man! W-O-M-A-N is spelled Double-You-Oh-Man!

Expecting men to react, feel and think the same way we women do, is just setting ourselves up for disappointment. We feel hurt when men don't live up to our unrealistic expectations. We get angry at them for being men, for a thousand things that men do or don't do, simply because they're men. When we react emotionally, remember we have sixteen times the impact, so when we blow up at them, or break into tears, men really don't want to, or can't, deal with it. This is frustrating for them, so they can get angry, and then we have a real fight on our hands.

But, you may be thinking, "Hold on a minute, does that mean it is the responsibility of the woman to adapt and adjust all the time? What about men doing their share?" Good point. However, think of it this way: Just as a computer can only print out what has been programmed in, men and women have been programmed to approach life differently. We each came from the Manufacturer with a special software package uniquely designed. It's nobody's fault! If you want to complain, talk to God, He's the Master Computer who designed us the way we are.

Woman is the embodiment of God's creative power. The word Shakti means "God's power in man-ifestation." Woman embodies the feminine aspect of God, through which "He" created the creation. That Primal Power is called the Adi Shakti and has been worshipped for centuries in the orient in the form of goddesses. Every woman has that divine goddess power in her own being, waiting to be recognized. Kundalini power is Shakti power.

EVERY WOMAN IS A GODDESS.

This is worth repeating:

EVERY WOMAN IS A GODDESS!

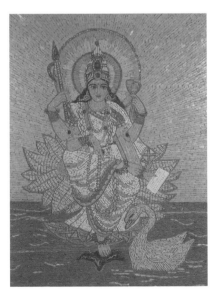

Saraswati, Goddess of Wisdom, Mother of Eloquence. Mosaic by Shakti Parwha Kaur Khalsa, 1967.

135

Yogi Bhajan's respect for women and his teachings are a reflection of Guru Nanak's words[3]:

"In a woman, we are conceived, and from a woman we are born
With a woman man is betrothed and married.
With a woman, man enjoys friendship and through a woman,
the path of life is created.
With a woman, man is engaged and married.
When woman has passed away, man seeks another woman.
To the woman, man is bound.
Why call that one bad from whom kings are born.
From a woman, a woman is born. Without a woman there can be none.
Nanak, only the one True Lord is without a woman..."

ACTION PLAN FOR WOMEN

(The following material is quoted directly from Yogi Bhajan's lectures.)

BE CALM, CONTENT, AND CONTAINED

"Never share your weaknesses with your man or your child. Go inside to your navel point, concentrate on it, and you'll get your answer in seconds. The only thing that can make you a failure in life is anxiety. Anxiety comes from the fact that your sense of achievement and sense of timing conflict. Learn to listen to others calmly and yourself quietly. The moment you don't listen to yourself, you will naturally become anxious. If you don't develop your personality so your presence will work, your words won't work either. Your presence should convince a person that he is talking to a goddess.

DISPOSABLE

"Life leaves very deep imprints on a woman. A lot of men try to use women as a toothpaste tube. They want her to be available when they want her, and when they are tired of her they replace her with a new one. A woman should understand her security before she indulges in relationships with men because all temporary relationships are very deeply imprinted on women. Men don't have that faculty, they are not affected the same way.

THE FLIRTATIOUS MIND

"There is a saying: 'There is a value for an arrogant mind but none for a flirtatious mind.' An arrogant mind is stubborn and demands information, whereas a flirtatious mind is self destructive. A mind which will

"A woman in America has only two choices: be a Goddess or be a prostitute." — Yogi Bhajan

destroy the self will destroy everything with it. A flirtatious mind is the worst thing which can happen to a woman. Unfortunately, because of her added mental faculty it is sometimes very easy for her to become flirtatious, as she does not know how to monitor herself. Once a woman has an aura of flirtatious behavior about her, it is very difficult for her to regain her respectability."

GGM: Grace of God Meditation

On September 22,1970, a group of women Kundalini Yoga students in San Francisco asked Yogi Bhajan how to control and channel their powerful, sometimes overwhelming emotions. They recognized that women do, indeed, have a lot to deal with! This was the day the GGM was born. For the first time, he taught the special meditation that is designed to awaken the power of the Adi Shakti, the goddess, within each woman. He called it the "Grace of God Meditation," "GGM" for short. You'll find it in the section called *Take Care of Yourself as a Woman* at the end of this book.

Women were not created to compete with men. Women were not intended to battle with men, but rather men and women were meant to complement and supplement each other.

What? No more battle of the sexes? Yes, the battle of the sexes can end. And it can end with a win/win situation, when we as women acknowledge and appreciate our power as women and use it positively.

MEN'S COURSES, Of Course!

For several years Yogi Bhajan taught courses especially for men, and even put some Men's Courses on video-tape. The Men's Courses were only for one day, whereas Women's Camp lasts several weeks each summer. He explained that women are far more complex than men, and in the long run, men would benefit more by his spending more time teaching the women how to be successful wives and mothers.

YOGI BHAJAN'S ADVICE TO MEN

"Whenever a woman cannot talk to you, raises her voice, or argues, she is covering her guilt. It has nothing to do with you. Her subconscious personality is reminding her of previous weaknesses which she doesn't want to fall into again. You are just a scapegoat. By faculty, she's not supposed to act that way. She is not talking to you, she is talking to her subconscious personality; she is in the past. Offer her a drink of water and change the subject."

WOMAN AS HER OWN PSYCHIATRIST

"The mental faculty of a female is multiple. Whereas a man can become 'singular,' this is impossible for a woman. By nature she is meant to protect a second life, that of her child. Nature has given her a subconscious, intuitive personality. Women have their outward personality and also this supplementary personality. But unfortunately the second personality, which is the added personality, creates a split personality.

"Something which was given to her as a gift to facilitate her motherhood, is becoming a psychiatric problem...The whole Western psychological and psychiatric world is totally baffled. They counsel woman without understanding that woman basically has no need to be counseled. She has to be awakened. No woman needs any advice and counseling. Woman can monitor herself, whereas man cannot."

HOW TO ANNOY A WOMAN

"You must understand that woman is much sharper than a male. No woman needs counseling. Her nature is to resist advice. If you want to annoy a woman, counsel her. She also gets angry more quickly than a man. A creature which can turn its blood into milk to save and nourish its offspring can do everything else also. A child can make a man crazy in ten minutes and not disturb a woman in twenty hours. The faculty of a woman also extends to mental and spiritual realms. She has an inborn capacity to tackle everything. She lives in the center of her being. Whereas by nature man either lives in his testicles or in his head. He does not have the natural tendency to live in the center of his being. But woman always lives in the center and works both up and down. There is a saying in the *Kama Shastra*, 'When a woman is in bed, sexual intercourse is perfect and she is totally blended with the man, even at that time she can think that the tea may boil over.' "

> **"Never underestimate the power of a woman."**
> — "Ladies Home Journal" Magazine Slogan

MARRIAGE

"MARRIAGE IS A CARRIAGE UNTO INFINITY"[4]

The divorce rate in America is astronomical, but if a woman understands the real purpose of marriage (instead of the fantasy about it) she has the ability to create a happy and successful relationship and a cozy home that a man will love to never leave. (Not that divorce is necessarily always the fault of the woman, but as they say, "Never underestimate the power of a woman.")

According to the highest spiritual understanding, marriage is a merger, an amalgamation of two souls out of which a new alloy is formed. When there are two bodies with one soul, it's a marriage. Wow! Talk about commitment!

A lot of books have been written about male female relationships and marriage, but Yogi Bhajan's teachings on the subject are startlingly different. They require a major re-evaluation of preconceived ideas. It's worth the effort, though. Women who have put these concepts into practice, have been helped to make dramatic changes in their lives.

"You all have to realize what a marriage is. Marriage is not an easy path. Marriage is a life. Marriage is not a ceremony, marriage is God.

"Marriage has not been understood by the Western world at all. It was understood by the Eastern world but it is forgotten there too. So at this time, the institution of marriage is in total limbo. People do not know what to do with

139

it; people do not know what to do without it. So what we have found out via the media is that marriage then divorce, and divorce then marriage, is a continuous process. But actually if we all understand what marriage is, then perhaps we can do better:

"Marriage is a partnership of two beings of light who live by their intuition, understanding, and a common, genuine interest of well being.

You are a help to each other. The purpose of the relationship is to relay the help. Rela-tion-ship: relay the ship. Deliver, deliver, deliver, deliver. It comes exactly to that..."

—Yogi Bhajan, KWTC June 29, 1988

"Marriage is an institution of willingness, in which two identities want to amalgamate. It's an amalgamation of two egos to bring out a neutral new personality.

"What is the advantage of it and what is the disadvantage of it? When this amalgamation happens then divine power in the psyche starts to function. Without that, people are individuals and they will only yell and scream at each other and goodness will never come in that home. It is a granted fact.

"Marriage brings happiness. It's an amalgamation of two psyches. And when these two psyches are amalgamated, neither one is an individual. There is no question of 'he' and 'she.'

"To make an alloy, you take two elements and put them together. The alloy cannot be separated. You can boil it, you can form the alloy into a liquid, you can totally burn it, but once it becomes an alloy, it will totally keep its own quality, own quantity, own weight, own molecules, own electrons, protons, and neutrons, and own combination. Whatever made brass doesn't matter. Brass has its own faculty, own quality, own weight, and own property. And that is what love is, that is what marriage is, that is what life is, that is what good luck is, when a male and a female merge together. That is why we marry before God."

As Yogi Bhajan says, "Everybody has faults. You divorce a man with 26 faults, but then you marry a man with a set of 27 other faults. What's the point? Broken hearts, broken homes. God lives in cozy homes, not in crazy homes." And it is the woman who creates the home, and it is the woman who becomes mother, the first teacher of our future generations.

TAKE IT LIGHTLY?

Today many people take marriage lightly, "Oh, if it doesn't work out, we'll get a divorce." And even having children is a pathetically casual affair. As Yogi Bhajan put it, "You take more care in preparing to plant a rose bush than you do to conceive a child." It is essential to understand that parents, and particularly the mother, play a most significant role in the shaping of the lifelong character, values, and attitudes of every generation. More about this in the *Four Teachers* Chapter.

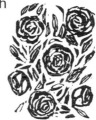

MOTHER'S 120th DAY

There is a beautiful custom of honoring a mother-to-be on the occasion of her 120th day of pregnancy. That is the day on which the soul actually enters the womb. Until the 120th day, according to ancient wisdom, there is really no "life" in the womb, only a piece of flesh, until the soul enters.

From the 120th day onward, the baby is receiving and absorbing input via the mother. What the mother hears, the baby hears; how the mother feels, the baby feels. What the mother says and does makes a distinct imprint on the child.

CHILD STAR

In her autobiography, *Child Star*, Shirley Temple Black, who was the most famous child motion picture star of all time, writes that her mother purposely went to museums, listened to beautiful music, read poetry, and even danced and sang while she was carrying Shirley, so that she would be sure to give birth to a talented, musically gifted child. In the *Mahabharata*[5] it speaks of the future warrior Arjuna being able to plan a successful battle strategy while still a young boy, because he remembered a conversation his father had with his mother while Arjuna was in her womb!

In 3HO, we have a big party to celebrate the mother's 120th Day. But it's not a baby shower. People bring gifts—but they're not for the baby, they are for the woman who is bringing a new life into the world. We honor her especially on this day, for she is the vehicle through which the the world receives a child who shall become a "saint, a hero, or a giver." That is the mother's assignment, to give the child spiritual values, so he can become that. And, all the time she must remember that the child does not belong to her, but belongs only to God. A child is no one's property.

PAY THE RENT

Being a parent is a job, and it's a challenging one. Parents are caretakers, teachers, and trainers. Parents are the ones who "pay the rent!" Kahlil Gibran's often quoted poem reminds us that our children don't belong to us. The attachment of parents to children, and its negative effects, is one of the hardest concepts for us to understand and accept - because we usually mistake attachment for love. It isn't. Learning the difference between mother love and "smother love" is one of our hardest lessons as women.

MANIFEST THE GODDESS ONE DAY AT A TIME

At the place where you relate to your Creator in the morning, place a sign that reads, "This Day Will I Be Graceful?" That day you will have to be graceful because you have asked the question and the answer is, "You will!" It should manifest in your way of speaking, eating, telephoning, behaving, taking a bath, dressing, driving a car, and so on. Your every action during that day must represent you as graceful. The most beautiful thing about it is that if you can do that for forty days, you will have achieved a state of mind in which little by little you can become totally perfect.

> "One thing every woman should know:
> SHOW NO INSECURITY.
> This is a key to royalty."
>
> —Yogi Bhajan

POWER OF A WOMAN

Guided Meditation for Women

"...See your power as a woman. Touch the heavens, squeeze it to yourself. Make all the oceans into just a drop. And out of this drop, you must squeeze all the stars and suns and moon. Beyond that, there is a space where you must excel. The gods shall listen to the call of the woman.

"The sound in the heavens, the murmur of the leaves; the music of the breeze; and the sound of the waves; the clouds in the skies and the dust on the earth - all in salutation to the call of the woman. The angels, divines, the sages, the saints are the existence of the very prayer of the woman. The calling of the 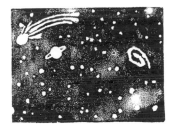 woman can penetrate through heavens and beyond all spaces into the infinity of God, and that's the only one power pure enough to manifest God on Earth..."

"...This is the truth. And you have to experience it. Woman is the only force. Living, vital, vibrating, her verbal sense is the only sense which is creative, which is consciousness..."

"...My dear children of God, there is a job to do. Put on your armor, alert yourself, and get going. The heavens shall bow to you. The angels will come. The demigods shall obey, and the Almighty God shall listen to you. Because you are the only way..."[6]

18
Four Teachers

Things Your Mother Never Told You

*U*nfortunately, most parents, including yours and mine, have to depend upon their instincts and the patterns they learned from their parents. Most of them are not yogis. They can only guide us within the limits of their own knowledge and experience. Even with the best of intentions, their own neuroses and biases color the way they teach us to deal with ourselves and the world.

Your first teacher in this school of life is your mother, second is your father, third is the environment (relatives, school teachers, friends), and finally, the fourth is your Spiritual Teacher whose job it is to correct any misconceptions you received from the first three.

It is not only what parents say to us, but what they do and what they are that deeply affects us and forms our basic attitudes toward ourselves and everyone else. We in turn pass along this legacy to our children, consciously or unconsciously.

MOTHER

Your first teacher is your mother. From the 120th day following conception (it is on the 120th day that the soul actually enters the womb) through the first three years of life, your mother's influence dominates. She is the primary, powerful, most compelling shaper of the attitudes, habits, prejudices, relationships, and self-images that usually stay with you for the rest of your life. For better or for worse, your mother's influence is almost indelible. The umbilical cord lasts well beyond the womb. The seeds of growing up with fear of failure, or fear of success, are planted during these early years.

FATHER

Your second teacher is your father. From age three to eight, his impact predominates. He is the male figure (or absence thereof) who supplies the example, the role model for a son. Dad is the archetype to imitate, to love, or to hate. Father personifies "man." For a daughter, Daddy or Poppa is the standard to which she will compare every other man she ever meets, for better or for worse.

RELATIVES and FRIENDS

The third teacher enters our consciousness at about age eight, in the form of brothers and sisters, relatives, neighbors, teachers, friends. They take on a major role of influence in our lives. Peer pressure rears its ugly head, and continues to grow stronger until it becomes enormous during the teen-age years. Of course, given ideal circumstances, peer pressure can be useful, supportive, and can encourage positive growth, but in most instances, it is the opposite.

SPIRITUAL TEACHER

The fourth teacher is your spiritual teacher. Most people born in the West don't really know what a "spiritual teacher" is. We suffer from a collective cultural deficiency, i.e., lack of education about the nature and function of a spiritual teacher and the necessity and importance of this relationship in our lives.

Who does he think he is? It's not a matter of "thinking," a genuine spiritual teacher KNOWS who he is. He has had the actual experience of confirming his identity beyond question. His mission in life is to help other people achieve that same experience. And when your soul leaves the body, he's there to help you make the transition. He works more in the non-physical planes than on the physical.

When you go mountain climbing, you hire a guide — someone who knows the way and the technology to get you to the top without falling and breaking your neck. He tells you where to step. You have the choice of following his instructions or not. You have that same choice on your spiritual path. Your spiritual teacher is like the rope with the hook on one end that you can safely climb up

Spirituality cannot be taught, it has to be caught, you have to get it from someone who's got it. That's why the inner connection with a spiritual teacher is so important.

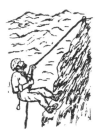

on, because it's anchored on the top. He offers himself as that rope. You have to project a link to it from your heart and then hold on! He takes on the weight of you and your karma as well as that of all the others he is helping to reach the same destination. That link is never broken by the teacher, but the student has the option to let go at anytime, and many do. It is that link of the mind and heart which we create with our teacher that enables him to help us free ourselves from our past, from our pain, from our patterns of fear, jealousy, greed, and anger, which cause us so much suffering and keep us trapped in our lower consciousness. Yogi Bhajan is my spiritual teacher.

Yogi Bhajan describes the student-teacher relationship:

Like a hammer and a chisel with a stone: when they meet, the sparks fly.

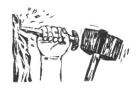

The relationship of a student to a spiritual teacher has to be described in analogies, because it is fundamentally so different from any other relationship you have. The relationship is not between personalities, although to the student it can appear to be!

A spiritual teacher is like a forklift who has to come down to earth, pick you up and lift you to the heights of his level of consciousness. When he meets you, how you perceive him depends upon your degree of consciousness. He can play whatever role you need in order for you to evolve.

TIME IS A TEACHER, TOO

Life is a school. We can choose: We can either learn our lessons in the hands of Time or from a Teacher. Our spiritual teacher acts as a catalyst to accelerate the learning process. He saves us time (perhaps even lifetimes). He doesn't necessarily make life easier, but he makes our growth as a spiritual being the main focus. He challenges us to fulfill our highest potential. He doesn't, and isn't supposed to, solve our problems for us, because that is OUR job. He gives us the tools and teaches us how to use them to cope with all the things we must face. He can suggest and recommend, but he cannot make our choices for us.

In this Aquarian Age, it is no longer adequate to know about something, we have to experience it. A spiritual teacher is not a preacher. Lots of people can give fabulous lectures and quote plenty of scripture. A spiritual teacher gives you an experience.

19
My Spiritual Teacher

YOGI BHAJAN

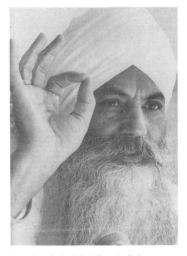

Siri Singh Sahib Bhai Sahib
Harbhajan Singh Khalsa Yogiji
also known as Yogi Bhajan

I thought I "knew it all" and I was not looking for a spiritual teacher when I met Yogi Bhajan. I was almost forty years old. I had been to India and had already studied with many other teachers. Some of what I had learned was wonderful and some of it was not. However, it was all valuable for it led me to the time and place where I could become Yogi Bhajan's student. Sooner or later, everyone gets one opportunity to meet their spiritual teacher. Not everyone recognizes nor accepts him. I almost missed my chance.

The day I met Yogi Bhajan, I privately told the woman who introduced us that I did not trust him. What I didn't know was that a real spiritual teacher is a mirror to our own consciousness. Come at him with your ego in full sail and you'll get zapped by the reflection of yourself right back at you - in no uncertain terms! Having been badly betrayed in the past by someone I had mistakenly regarded as a spiritual teacher, I was full of skepticism. (And pretty full of myself!) Fortunately, I was strongly impressed by the depth of love and light I saw in the eyes of this courtly mannered, soft spoken yogi.

A true spiritual teacher has already experienced the state of "yoga," or divine union with his own infinity. He recognizes that same, divine identity in every other human being. Therefore, he truly loves and accepts everyone. These authentic spiritual teachers, "masters," "saints," yogis, come to wake us up to

149

reality. They usually shake us up in the process. They challenge us, they teach us, and they pray for us. Their mission is to enable us to experience our true

You are not a human being having a spiritual experience; you are a spiritual being having a human experience.

identity as divine beings in human form. They are often crucified for this attempt.

It was December 22, 1968, at a lecture at the East West Cultural Center that I first met Yogi Bhajan. After the program, a small group of us went out to dinner together, including "the yogi." I was quite surprised when he suddenly leaned forward from the other end of the table and said, "Your son's in trouble, isn't he? I can help you." I didn't know what to make of this strange tall man, with such a striking appearance. Since my son was indeed in serious trouble, I didn't want to pass up any opportunity for help. So, just a few days later, on Christmas day, I phoned Yogi Bhajan and went to see him. He not only told me the story of his life, he also told me the story of my life!

The ability to see into a person's innermost being, to know what that soul has experienced, as well as to see its destiny, is one of the major attributes of a spiritual teacher. Yogi Bhajan's vision is not limited to outer appearances.

This is what he told me: He had been hired to teach Kundalini Yoga at Toronto University, but the day before his plane from New Delhi landed, the head of the department who had hired him was killed in an auto accident. The job was no longer there. To make matters worse, his luggage had been lost en route. Of course he had been warned by the pandits and astrologers in India that he should wait until a more auspicious time to make the trip. They had told him he would have a very hard time in the West unless he postponed his departure. But as we have learned through the years, it is not in Yogi Bhajan's nature to retreat from difficulty. He confronts challenge head on. He listens to everyone's advice, but he always acts according to his own inner guidance.

In Canada, he was really a stranger in a strange land, dealing with a very different culture. The cold Canadian winter had just set in. He had to tie newspapers around his shoes to keep warm. He didn't know where his next meal was coming from. Sometimes it didn't come. Then he got a job working as a shipping clerk in a book store. When he was invited to come to Los Angeles for a weekend, he gladly accepted. That's when I met him. After our conversation on December 25th, I offered to drive him to an appointment the next day. That is when he gave me the mantra that changed my life.

He explained to me that nothing in this world is more powerful than the prayer of a mother for her son. He wrote down the words **EK ONG KAR SAT NAM SIRI WHA GURU** on a little piece of paper. He told me that if I would chant this mantra powerfully from the navel point, all in one breath, for one hour every day before sunrise and pray for my son, he would be all right. (At the time I didn't even know where my son was, only that he had attempted suicide and gone A.W.O.L. from the United States Army.)

I already had a spiritual routine I was doing daily, including several other mantras. When Yogi Bhajan gave me this one, I asked him, "What about all the other things I'm doing?" (Sufi chanting, Hopi Indian mantra, and Vedanta meditation.) He said, "Go ahead and do everything, but try this also."

That seemed reasonable to me, so that's what I did. On the second day of chanting, I had such a profound experience that I could barely wait until I could phone him and say, "I don't have to do anything else, this is it." Now, twenty-seven years later, although we chant many other mantras that Yogi Bhajan has taught us, those syllables are still "mine."

(I am happy to say that within ten days I heard from my son. He had been "rescued" up in Berkeley, which is a whole story in itself, with no space in this book for it! We were able to work things out with the army. I'm also happy to say that I saved the precious piece of paper on which Yogi Bhajan wrote those eight magic words. It's carefully preserved in my scrapbook of the early days of 3HO.)

Yogi Bhajan had told me during my first interview with him, "You have been a student long enough, you should be a teacher." He said that he had come to train teachers, not to get disciples. At the time I thought to myself, "Oh, sure, fat chance." He said although I knew a lot, he could "put it all together for me." I thought, "Who does he think he is?"

I found out! He is an amazing living phenomenon of perpetual creativity. When he lectures, a spontaneous flow of divine inspiration comes through him. Put him in any situation, he will always attune himself to the needs of that particular group of people, time, and place. Yogi Bhajan is the pipeline, the "postman" delivering the divine message that each of us is a soul, our identity is Truth (**SAT NAM**) and we're here to experience That. He tells us that it is foolish and a mistake to worship the messenger, but I have observed it is equally foolish to ignore the message!

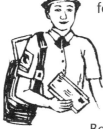

Where Yogi Bhajan is concerned, throw out your preconceived ideas of what a spiritual teacher is. Part of the job he does so masterfully is to confuse your intellect so that you have to go beyond your mind. God cannot be experienced so long as our perception is limited within the confines of the intellect.

Because he is a Teacher, Yogi Bhajan gives tests constantly. He often uses the "poke, provoke, confront, and elevate" technique. He pushes us to break out of the confinement of our limited little egos. This does not necessarily make him popular. In fact we (our egos, that is) can definitely resent what he says. Truth about ourselves is often hard to swallow much less digest.

I've never met anyone so adept at "pushing my buttons" as Yogi Bhajan. But, alas, I know that so long as I have buttons that can be pushed, I'm still living in my ego and reacting, and that blocks my own spiritual growth.

Sometimes the test is simply to recognize that what he says, or the situation we are in, is a test! Test of what? Those qualities we need to learn in order to graduate from this earth school-of-life: non-attachment, patience, faith, kindness, obedience, surrender to the will of God, humility.

Each of us is different, each of us has a unique curriculum to master. Therefore, the spiritual teacher provides a specialized tutorial for every individual under his direct guidance, plus he has to provide universal guidelines and principles that apply to everyone. Yogi Bhajan's teachings are based on such universal Truths.

To many people in the '60s and '70s Yogiji became the father figure. Lovingly, patiently, humorously, he cajoled, encouraged, helped, and inspired a whole generation to try Kundalini Yoga instead of drugs. He never said, "No," or "Don't" do this or that, he gave alternatives. He taught three classes, six days a week, and a meditation class on Sundays for over a year.

Meanwhile, he was studying our culture, our attitudes, our personal histories of abuse and neglect, betrayal, and abandonment. Out of his compassion he began to create more opportunities for us to heal and strengthen ourselves. He created 3HO events such as Summer and Winter Solstice Sadhanas, and Khalsa Women's Training Camp (KWTC). In 1970, when he became the Mahan Tantric, he put himself on the line even more, taking on more stress by allowing anyone and everyone to participate in the White Tantric Yoga group meditation courses he taught. *(See the chapter Tantric Yoga.)*

Through the years he has given us many insights into his personal philosophy of life. Here's one such gem:

FIVE CORNERSTONES OF YOGI BHAJAN'S STRENGTH

1. Never let out that which can harm anyone.
2. Never let in what can harm you.
3. Never let down friend or foe.
4. Light up that corner where no one has the courage.
5. Keep up and keep the harmony.

Perhaps you have never met Yogi Bhajan. But I assure you, if you are practicing Kundalini Yoga, and certainly if you are teaching it, it is his mastery that supports your spiritual growth. He and all the spiritual teachers who have preceded him, are called into service whenever you chant **ONG NAMO GURU DEV NAMO**. It is not the people, but their spiritual consciousness, their subtle bodies, who are with you, like guardian angels invoked by those syllables.

THE GOLDEN CHAIN

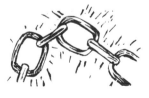

Through the ages, the transference of spiritual awareness, consciousness, and power has been handed down from master to disciple, in a continuous chain whose links are forged of reverence, obedience, devotion, and humility on the part of the student, and infinite love and sacrifice on the part of the teacher. This ongoing connection is sometimes called the "golden chain."

MAHAN TANTRIC

Yogi Bhajan is unique among spiritual teachers because he is also the Mahan Tantric of this era. This means that he is the only living master of White Tantric Yoga in the world, since there can only be one on the planet at any given time. He is a world teacher, a very special instrument whom God has appointed and anointed to awaken the millions of sleeping souls on this planet.

He is a Teacher of teachers. His words have enormous power. His being vibrates in harmony with the universal consciousness and he feels everything before it happens. He cannot compromise the integrity of his responsibility as a teacher, so he cannot tell all that he knows. His power is not his own, and he knows it. He says his power is his own inner prayer, which is calm, quiet, and peaceful. (Though outwardly, most students will attest, his energy comes across like a tornado!)

GO CLIMB A TREE?

Yogi Bhajan tells a great story about one of the ways Sant Hazara Singh, his Kundalini Yoga teacher in India (and the Mahan Tantric during those years), tested him. Wearing his best starched clothes and shined shoes, he was traveling with his teacher to meet some dignitary. Sant Hazara Singh told the driver to stop the car, and instructed young Harbhajan Singh to get out. He pointed to a nearby tree and told him to climb it, and to stay there until he came back. As a good student, the boy didn't ask why, he didn't hesitate. He got out, climbed the tree and waited. His teacher drove off. Three days and nights went by. He stayed up in that tree! When his teacher finally came back and released him, he never asked him how he had managed, never congratulated him on his obedience and resourcefulness. The matter was never discussed. Of course that was in India, where they understand what it means to serve a spiritual teacher, and what can be gained. Yogi Bhajan knew the rules of the relationship: never ask why, never deny, simply say "Yes, Sir," and do it. God only knows what one of us would do under similar circumstances.

A spiritual teacher never settles for anything less than the best from a student. His job is not to praise us when we do well, but to present the next lesson immediately so we can continue to grow. He can never be satisfied.

Yogi Bhajan has told us many stories about his experiences as a student. One of them is about a time when he was a young military officer, already quite an accomplished yogi. However, he wanted to learn a particular kriya from a teacher whom he had never met. Every day he would go to pay his respects, hoping for an audience. The teacher ignored him for months. Then he sent word that he should personally prepare and bring a carrot pudding as an offering every day. He also insisted that Harbhajan walk the five miles to get there. This went on for months before the teacher would even talk to him. The young military officer, in his immaculately starched and pressed uniform had to leave his car and his driver behind, and make the trek barefoot, carrying that carrot pudding. He did it. Would you?

In the West, we have not been taught to respect the cosmic laws which govern the student—teacher relationship. In fact, most people don't even know what they are. So, in our ignorance, we are not able to take full advantage of the benefits and blessings a teacher can offer. It is also true that there has been exploitation and abuse of the role of Spiritual Teacher by people claiming to be "enlightened." Before you get involved with any teacher, you should investigate this area for yourself. Come to your own conclusions. I learned about spiritual teachers through reading and through trial and error during fifteen years of exploring various spiritual paths before I met Yogi Bhajan. One thing I know for sure, watch out for any teacher who wants you to worship him. If you consider someone your spiritual teacher, he deserves your utmost respect and reverence. If he or she is a genuine Teacher, and you want to excel, give your obedience. For those who are destined to lead must first learn to follow. But always remember, the teacher is the guide, not the destination.

TEACHER OF TEACHERS

True to his word, Yogi Bhajan has trained hundreds of teachers of Kundalini Yoga. The 3HO Foundation, (Healthy, Happy, Holy Organization) which he founded in 1969, is a teacher training organization with centers all over the world. He told us:

155

"If you want to learn something, read about it. If you want to understand something, write about it. If you want to master something, teach it." He wants us all to be masters. He tells us to be "ten times greater" than he is. And he means it.

He also warned all of us who were to become teachers that, "You will be tested in three areas: money, sex, or power—possibly in all of them." It is a great responsibility and privilege to teach Kundalini Yoga. It is said that if a teacher betrays the sacred trust placed in him, he will be reborn as a cockroach!

"Don't serve lineage, serve legacy."
—Yogi Bhajan

YOGI BHAJAN'S POETRY AND ART

The Siri Singh Sahib, Yogi Bhajan has written many, many poems. A special collection has been published in a book called *Furmaan Khalsa*. Many of his poems have been set to music and are on tape. He has painted pictures, designed jewelry, and gathered together a magnificent collection of statuary, paintings and other art objects all of which he has donated to the Sikh Dharma archives. A museum is planned to house these treasures.

BIOGRAPHY OF A YOGI

Born August 26, 1929, in the village of Kot Harkaran, now in Pakistan, Harbhajan Singh Puri was the son of a medical doctor and a very devout and powerful mother. He mastered Kundalini Yoga when he was sixteen. Still only a teenager when India was partitioned, he took charge of leading a thousand people out of his village to safety near New Delhi. During his youth he studied with many teachers, including his revered grandfather, Bhai Fateh Singh, and the Mahan Tantric, Sant Hazara Singh. He attended Punjab University where he majored in Economics, was an all-around athlete, and a champion debater. I have his prize certificates in my files. Captain of the soccer team, track star, he used his Kundalini Yoga practice to get in shape for athletic events. He was a winner!

He married Inderjit Kaur, and they had three children (and now five grandchildren born in the United States). He was a Commanding Officer in the Indian Army, starting out in the Motor Transport division, and he served in the Indian Government for eighteen years before coming to America.

Harbhajan Singh Khalsa Yogiji became a United States citizen in 1976 and earned his Ph.D. in psychology in 1980. His doctoral dissertation is called "Communication, Liberation or Condemnation."

His bottom line is:

Understand the fact that God is in all, big and small.

His motto is:

If You Can't See God In All, You Can't See God At All

20
Communication

After years of ministerial counseling I have come to the conclusion that most problems between people are problems in communication. Yes, of course we all have our neuroses, and trust is a major issue, but when two people really communicate with each other, a lot of problems can be solved. Even wars eventually have to go to the negotiating table to finalize peace. Why not start there?

There is a whole science to effective communication so that your words will be received and understood the way you intend them. Yogi Bhajan's doctoral dissertation titled: "Communication, Liberation or Condemnation," is on this very subject. It goes into great detail about the use of the various chakras (energy centers) in communication.

"Communication is very misunderstood by all human beings

When you are angry,
When you are emotional,
When you are hurt,
When you are insecure.

Or when you are into an ego trip —
That's when you feel you must talk,
And that's why you mess up!

Because when you talk it should be for the future, not for the past or the present. Communication is the art of building heaven in the future."[1]

YOGI BHAJAN SPEAKS ABOUT WORDS and CHAKRAS:

"...What should I say? The two most important things in your body are the upper palate, which is the base of the hypothalamus, and the tip of the tongue. Every word spoken by you is made with the palate and the tongue in combination with the hypothalamus, which controls the entire neurons of the brain. The tongue has a central nervous system controlling your total psyche. You can change the whole world with the word. World is dependent on the word. W-O-R-D and W-O-R-L-D. The central nervous system, shushmana, is at the tip of the tongue. And your entire neuron section is up here under the hypothalamus where the stimulation of the eighty-four meridian points takes place. It's decided by the permutation and combination. But there is a chakra involved. Ask me any question, I'll tell you which chakra will answer what.

Q: What is the difference between communicating from the fifth center and the sixth center?

A: With any communication, one center is involved. You have to decide what the purpose is. If the purpose is to mess up somebody, go with the first chakra. If you want to seduce somebody, go with the second. If you want to balance out somebody, go with the third. If you want to uplift somebody, go with the fourth. If you want to be blunt, go by the fifth. If you want to command somebody and take the responsibility and see it is done and delivered, then go by the sixth. If you want to just get rid of somebody, go by the seventh. You know what the seventh is? 'I see the light in you better than me. God bless you, you are wonderful.' The guy will shut up in two minutes."

SPEAKING OF SPEAKING:

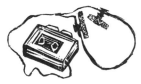

Did you ever analyze how much of what you say is encouraging, uplifting, and positive — and how much is not? Much of our ordinary, every day conversation is negative and self-negating. We barely notice the destructive nature of the words we use because the "put-down" is so common in our society.

Start listening to your words. If you really want to have an adventure, tape record yourself for a whole day and then listen to what you have said. You'll be shocked, especially when you remember you are "creating" whenever you speak. The old admonition to "think before you speak" is still good advice. It's easier to do that when you have your nerves under control. Nerves have to be very strong so you don't automatically react to everything that happens the minute it happens, like a robot responding to a button being pushed. *(I hope you read the chapter called Stress, Stamina, and Nerves of Steel.)*

Another fascinating experiment in self-awareness is to go on silence for a few days. It can be quite a revelation. I've done it. It was very humbling. If you really do it, you'll probably discover as I did, how much conversation is not really necessary or useful at all (including your own!).

In the *Things To Do* section you'll find two meditations Yogi Bhajan taught specifically to help us improve our communication.

CHOOSE YOUR WORDS

Words are the colors
On the speaker's palate
Evoking emotion
In the ear of the beholder

Some are dull and some are bright
Some are wrong and some are right
Some ennoble and some degrade
One Word created this creation
...   So it was said

Be Careful
Be Courageous
Be Conscious
Be sure
Before you speak—
Will your words kill — or cure?

Words can comfort
Words can enrage
Words can liberate
Or words can cage
Some
> *Words are weapons*
> *Words are bandages*
> *Words are penicillin*
> *Words are poison*

Words are hot
And words are cold
Words speak Truth —
With words, lies are told

162

Honor your words
Use your words with honor
For words can heal
Or words can kill

Aim your words with extra care
Lasers pierce targets everywhere
Relationships built over many years
One false word dissolve in tears

Words reveal
And words hide
True Identity
Divine inside

Faith in the Word
Dispels all fear
Hold your words gently
Hold your words dear
Be honest, be kind
Make yourself clear

To belittle is common
To uplift is rare
Value your words
Use them with care

Power to speak comes from breath of life
Surgeon's scalpel or butcher knife
Speak to your soul with respect in place
You'll speak to others with equal grace.

The Snake That Poisons Everybody[3]

It
topples
governments,
wrecks
marriages,
ruins
careers,
busts
reputations,
causes
heartaches,
nightmares,
indigestion,
spawns suspicion,
generates
grief,
dispatches
innocent
people
to cry in their
pillows.
Even its name
hisses.
It's called
gossip.
Office gossip,
Shop gossip,
Party gossip.
It makes
headlines
and headaches.
Before
you repeat
a story,
ask yourself:
Is it true?
Is it fair?
Is it necessary?
If not,
shut up.

How we perform as individuals will
determine how we perform as a nation.

21
Happiness

Everyone wants to be happy. At least consciously. The problem is in the subconscious. Subconsciously some of us may not be ready to give up our suffering. Some of us are so used to feeling miserable that we don't know who we'd be if we stopped feeling sorry for ourselves!

What would we have to talk about if we quit complaining? Dr. Donald Curtis (Science of Mind minister) used to call it the "P.L.O.M." syndrome. "Poor Little Old Me" is a pretty common self-image in our society. It doesn't lend itself to happiness. Some people's self image is so tied up with feeling victimized, or feeling "unworthy" that they can't even imagine what it would be like to be happy. Yet happiness is the birthright of every human being. The true nature of the soul is joy!

Happiness goes way beyond pleasure or enjoyment. Happiness is an inner state of being. It comes when we are in touch with the permanent part of ourselves, the God within us, that is always in bliss. The essential nature of God is described by Vedanta philosophy as "Sat, Chit, Anand": Truth, Knowledge, and Bliss.

Happiness is NOT dependent upon any outside person, event, or thing.

We are each responsible for our own happiness. It is how I personally choose to relate to a person, event, or thing; the kind of thought, feeling, or emotion that I choose to hold about it, that determines my happiness or unhappiness. I can't blame anyone else for how I feel about my life. If I view what's happening from the telescope of the divine consciousness within me, I'll have a different experience than if I look at it with the microscope of my personal emotions. Happiness is a state of being. Happy or unhappy is how I "am."

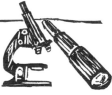

"Happiness runs in a circular motion,
 Life is like a little boat upon the sea,
 Everybody is a part of everything anyway,
 You can have it all if you let yourself be..."
—Donovan

Happiness comes from giving, and having an attitude of gratitude. Happiness has to do with being god-like. That's not asking too much, since the core identity of each of us is Spirit. That's why these Seven Steps To Happiness apply:

The Seven Steps to Happiness

The seven steps to happiness are: commitment, character, dignity, divinity, grace, power to sacrifice, experience of happiness. There is no other way you can be happy. Here's how Yogi Bhajan elaborated on them at KWTC, 1989.

1. **COMMITMENT:** to kindness and to compassion, it gives you character.

2. **CHARACTER:** is a pattern of behavior where you can clearly answer and stand before your own consciousness, it leads to Dignity.

3. **DIGNITY:** is when you act as a god for another, then you gain Divinity.

4. **DIVINITY:** is when you put yourself and your life on the line to serve another person or a creature, which leads you to Grace.

5. **GRACE:** is when you've developed a presence that works so that you have the Power to Sacrifice.

6. **POWER TO SACRIFICE:** is when God sits in your heart and presides in your head and you can therefore sacrifice — and that takes you to Happiness.

7. **HAPPINESS:** is when you can be thankful for the chance of being these seven things.

22

THE WORLD ACCORDING TO ME, with a little help from Vedanta Philosophy and a few other teachings:

Life is a Movie

In 1943, when I was thirteen, my mother and I moved to the entertainment capital of the world, HOLLYWOOD, CALIFORNIA! It was the Golden Age of film. Everybody went to the movies regularly. I still do. I love to be entertained, don't you? That's why we go to the movies, read books and plays, and watch television. We're fascinated, intrigued, inspired, frightened, or amused by the tales we hear or see. We can experience all sorts of adventures vicariously. The best teachers and public speakers are the ones who are good story tellers. They entertain us. Here's a good story for you:

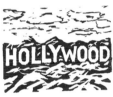

"Once upon a time, before time began..." according to Vedanta philosophy, God created this entire creation. It is said He did it for His entertainment, so this whole creation is known as God's "Leela," His "play." Everything we see around us is part of His story, unfolding for His entertainment!

I figure that must be why we, His creatures, made by Him, "in His image," enjoy stories (substitute "movies" here) so much. It's because we're "God-like"!

As I understand it, God was just kind of sitting around, not doing much of anything, simply existing as a vast, shoreless ocean of existence, absolutely silent and still. Static. No ripples, no movement, no activity. Just a vast expanse of "being" — a timeless, beginningless, and endless ocean with no surface and no bottom. In other words, unmanifest, infinite, unlimited in any way. Then at one unmeasurable point, God set into motion within Himself, a vibration that created ripples and waves. In other words, God "spoke." With one mighty roar, He created the creation. He made Himself colder in some places, forming icebergs; and hotter in others, forming steam; He laughed and played, watching and experiencing the interaction of Himself with Himself in a tremendous variety of

167

shapes, and forms, and colors all taking place within, and composed of the ocean of His own Being-ness. His story became manifest.

Describing or imagining God as an ocean is, of course, just one of many analogies people have used to try to understand what God is. At least for me, the ocean analogy works. It makes it easier to understand how God can be, and is always, everything and everywhere. I repeat:

God is everything that ever was, is now, or shall ever be.

"Aad Such,
Jugaad Such,
Habhee Such,
Nanak Hosee Bhee Such..."
True in the beginning,
True through all the ages,
True even now,
Nanak[1] says Truth shall exist forever.

RULES OF THE GAME

Let's go back to the analogy of God as an ocean of existence that created a game (out of the "water"of His own being) of shapes and forms that interact with each other. It's the game of life. And God created a whole system of evolution within this game. Just as a child at play builds a sand castle and then knocks it over and builds it up all over and over again, God Generates, Organizes, and then Destroys (or Delivers) everything within His Creation.

He made the planets and the stars, earth, and sky, and oceans (wet ones), rivers, lakes, and trees, and birds, and you, and me. And He made rules for His Game. These are called cosmic laws. They include the law of karma. Karma is automatic. It is based on the principle of action and reaction. The way it works is sometimes described as "As you sow, so shall you reap." We get back what

168

we send out, and that's a fact. However, it may take many lifetimes to get all the results — or reactions — from the actions we have set into motion, until everything gets finally balanced out.

Nobody really ever "gets away with" anything, even though it may seem like it. Karma has to be paid, if not now, later; perhaps in a next lifetime. Sooner or later "what goes around comes around." However, with the blessing of God and the grace of the Guru, karma can be softened by Dharma (path of righteousness/spiritual path). Your spiritual teacher can also help by taking on some of the karma your soul agreed to pay off in this lifetime. He can counsel you and guide you to make the decisions that will most effectively fulfill your destiny and teach you the lessons you came to this planet to learn. The spiritual teacher can save you lots of time and useless suffering if you're smart enough to listen carefully to him. Another analogy: Life is a school.

SCENE: Schoolroom called Earth

Everyone gets challenges and tests, because Earth is a school, and we have come here to learn the lessons our souls need in order to graduate. (This is part of the script God wrote.)

Either we learn in the hands of Time or from a Spiritual Teacher.

Your soul agreed to be born at a certain time and place (yes, you chose your own parents), with the scenery, cast, and crew chosen to support you in your starring role in your personal story. The folks closest to you are most likely people who have some strong karmic connection to you from the past.

(We're back to the movie analogy:)

This "movie" is God's game of life. It's God's show. God is playing all of the roles. He is actually all of the actors and actresses! He is the author, the screen writer, director, and producer, as well as the scenery and the audience. God is even the ticket-taker, the usher, and the boy who sells the popcorn!

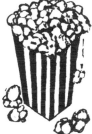

THE SHOW MUST GO ON

When scientists split the atom back in the '40s, the energy that was released was, and still is, the very same energy that the yogis have known about and played with for thousands of years. They call it "prana." It is the incoming life breath. It is prana that God puts into you every time He gives you another breath of life. Each time you inhale it is God breathing the essence of Himself into you so that His show can go on. Maybe that's where the saying, "The show must go on!" originated.

Choose the analogy you like, "ocean, movie, game." In any case, life is happening, and we are acting (or reacting) in its story, playing the roles we were given. The thing is, someday the show will be over and we must go Home. Going "Home" means going back to GOD, from Whom we came in the first place. Winning the game of life means going home consciously. Consciously expanding your self-awareness until you remember, recognize, and experience that you are the whole ocean. "You and God, God and you are ONE." That experience of your own identity is the ultimate goal of practicing yoga. It is the goal of all human existence.

"All things come from God, and all things go to God."[2] (There's no place else to go!)

Here comes a really long sentence: When we die, all we are doing is taking off the costume that we wore in this show, and leaving it behind in this theater called earth so we can return to the absolute freedom, joy and bliss of the vastness of the ocean of God, which is so marvelously fantastic and wonderful, that for those who have had this experience, all they can say in trying to describe it, is "Wahe Guru!" which means "Wow! God is great beyond description."

Meanwhile, while we're playing our roles in these bodies, it's God's intention for us to enjoy it. That's why He created it in the first place, remember? "Leela" means play! (Schools have playgrounds, too, and even classrooms can be fun for good students.)

If we're not enjoying life, it's because we've forgotten that life is a movie and we're taking our roles too seriously. If we're not happy, it's because we're stuck in our lower chakras (*Energy centers. See chapters Mysterious Kundalini and*

170

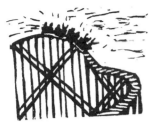

Chakras) and not utilizing our higher consciousness. If we're listening to our minds instead of our intuition, if we're emotional and commotional — riding the roller coaster of emotional turmoil and reacting to situations instead of resurrecting, we're most likely not happy campers!

Which leads us back to Kundalini Yoga. It's a technology to enable us to control our emotions and minds (not suppress or deny them, but take charge of them, ruling kindly but firmly over them, rather than being a slave to them) so we can enjoy the drama, the comedy. We can go through any tragedy in life without letting it overwhelm us or destroy our happiness.

Happiness, after all, really lies within, not outside ourselves. My reality, my happiness or unhappiness, is what I choose to feel within my own being, and it can't be dependent upon any outside influence. The inherent nature of the soul is joyful. When I'm in tune with, in touch with, in synch with my soul, I'm bound to be happy! Activating the Kundalini so that it can function in the higher chakras makes it much more conveniently possible to do that.

When circumstances are not pleasant, I try to remind myself that life is, after all, a movie. I want to enjoy the film, whether it's a comedy or a tragedy. And I want to remember that some day the lights will go on, the projector will be turned off, and we'll all go Home!

SHOPPING FOR HIGHER CONSCIOUSNESS (another analogy)

You've gone to buy linens in your favorite department store. You push the elevator button to go up to seven, but on the third floor, the elevator stops, the doors open briefly, and your eye catches sight of something really irresistible and appealing. You decide you'll step off for "just a quick look." You find more and more to look at, and get so totally absorbed in browsing through all the fascinating things — lots of them on sale, too (!), — that you lose track of time, and forget the original mission that brought you to the store. By that time the store has closed and you're trapped. It's called "maya." Similarly, it's easy to get trapped in "spiritual maya." Occult powers and psychic phenomena are examples of spiritual maya.

171

All the distractions in our lives are maya. In Sanskrit, "maya" literally means "that which can be measured." It is the polarity to the infinite. Maya is understood in Vedanta philosophy as the "apparent creation." All that 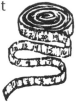 we can see and hear and touch and taste with our five senses, anything measurable in any way, is maya. It can be fascinating, it is enticing, it can be fun, but it is not permanent. It can't last forever. There's nothing "wrong" with maya. It can give lots of pleasure and excitement, but maya cannot provide happiness. Happiness comes only from within, nowhere else. When you touch that reality of God within you, that is happiness.

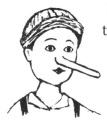 Like Pinocchio being lured away to the fair instead of going to school, the glitter of maya can make us forget where we're going, too! So, before we invest a lot of time and energy in anything, any person, or any activity, it makes good sense to ask ourselves, "Is this really the best use of my time? How much of a detour can I afford to take? Will this really take me towards Home, or farther away?"

BUBBLES AND BRIDGES

"I am the bubble, make me the sea
I am the bubble, make me the sea
So do Thou my Lord, make me the sea, oh make me the sea
Thou and I are never apart, Thou and I are never apart..."

In the early days after Yogi Bhajan's arrival in America, I used to sing this song from the Self-Realization Fellowship song book. He really liked it. Bubbles, sea — it fits right in with the ocean analogy.

Analogies are sometimes useful, but they're limited. They are intellectual attempts to clarify ideas, concepts that can't totally be grasped by the intellect. They do give us a bridge of understanding. But to really cross over the bridge, we can't just talk about getting to the other side. We have to do something. There's a big difference between describing water and drinking it, or actually jumping in the ocean and swimming! What to do, and how to do it, the ways and means to get your own direct experience of God or Truth, is what Yoga is all about.

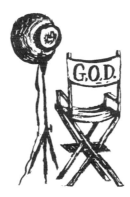

PAST LIVES

In what lifetime did we meet?
For what reason did we part?
Did you — or did I — break somebody's heart?

What job is ours?
What lessons to learn?
What debt to pay?
What credit to earn?

Do we clash today
Because of wounds long ago?
Were we friends or lovers?
(Would it help to know?)

Past lives' fascination
Pulls our focus off track
We need to look forward —
Not go back

Whatever was then
Brought us to now
The riddle of life
To solve somehow

This time do it right
Once and for all
Climb the heights
No more to fall

Look to the Light
Open your heart
Master's touch
Gives a head start

Truth beyond time
Love beyond space
Infinite souls
Meet in this place.

(I wrote this poem while facilitating
White Tantric Yoga in Espanola, New
Mexico, Nov. 30, 1991)

23
Other Paths of Yoga

For those readers who are not familiar with the various paths of yoga, here are some brief descriptions:

Hatha Yoga is the most well-known yoga. It is a beautiful discipline for strengthening the body, with emphasis on developing the will. It utilizes eighty-four traditional yogic postures (asanas) and uses various breathing techniques (pranayam). Practice of Hatha Yoga requires patience and emphasizes flexibility. Mastery takes many years.

Bhakti Yoga is the path of devotion, in which the student or devotee focuses on a particular deity and offers all his or her actions out of love to that "Beloved." Chanting God's name, reciting hymns in praise of God, remembering God, surrendering, worshipping God in a personalized form is the way of the Bhakti yogi.

Karma Yoga is the path of the man or woman of action. (Mahatma Gandhi was an adherent of Karma Yoga.) It requires one to surrender the fruits of one's actions to God. The Karma Yogi always keeps in mind that God is truly the Doer of everything. Therefore, the results of any action do, in fact, belong to Him (He/She/It: GOD). Such non-attachment to the results of one's actions frees a person from creating more karma. An analogy often given for non-attachment is "to live in the world but not of it," or to "be like the lotus in the pond," whose beautiful white blossom remains pure and unstained above the water, unaffected by the mud clinging to its roots below.

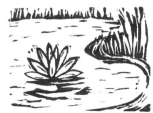

175

Gyan Yoga is considered the path of the intellect, which is by nature a divisive instrument, always separating and comparing. The Gyan Yogi might spend his whole life looking at the Creator and the creation as separate, which would account for the usual textbook description "not this, not that." People sometimes think that Buddha denied the existence of God because he would never say what God is. I think Buddha just didn't want to limit God by trying to define or describe Him.

The intellect is a limited tool. Language can only take us so far. Words can motivate and inspire, uplift and create, but we have go beyond words, beyond intellectual understanding, to have the direct personal experience of merging with God. That merger is sometimes called "Divine Union." It is "Yoga." You not only get to New York, you become New York! By the way, I do not consider reaching New York the ultimate goal of life. This is just an analogy. God does, of course, live everywhere, including New York.

TRI-MARGA

The Bhagavad Gita *(See the Recommended Reading List)* calls Karma Yoga, Bhakti Yoga and Gyan Yoga the "Tri-Marga" or Threefold Path.

Raj Yoga is the Royal path, whose method has been preserved in the written aphorisms of Patanjali. These aphorisms have been translated and commented upon in wonderful detail by Christopher Isherwood and Swami Prabhavananda in the book, *How to Know God* (high on my recommended reading list). The eight steps on the path to liberation or Samadhi begin with ethical precepts, the "do's" and "don'ts" by which the aspirant guides his life. They are called *Yams* and *Niyams*. Then Raj Yoga defines and describes the postures (*Asanas*); the place where the yogi sits, and how he sits; breathing techniques (*Pranayam*); becoming aware of and controlling the thought waves in the mind (*Pratyahar*).

Pratyahar is the great-grandfather of positive thinking. It utilizes the technique of substituting a positive vibration in the mind for a negative one. Concentration (*Dharana*); meditation (*Dhyana*); and absorption in God (Liberation or *Samadhi*) are the final steps.

176

Patanjali also wrote about the nature of the mind and the ego, the various types of purification needed to follow the path of Raj Yoga, and the powers that can come along with its practice.

Mantra Yoga is exactly what the name implies, a path of chanting and meditating on sacred syllables, raising one's vibration through the repetition of sound current. If you think about a drop of water taking a few centuries to make a dent in a rock, you can understand why mantras are repeated over and over again. In some cases it takes a lot of time and repetition to make a change in our consciousness! There are several kinds of sound which are described in detail in our chapter on Mantra.

Laya Yoga may be considered the post-graduate program in Mantra Yoga. It is a more sophisticated use of sound, taking mantra another step further.

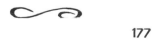

24
Tantric Yoga

"There's a difference like day and night between the three types of tantric. They are totally different. They are definitely different in quality, quantity, direction, practices, methods, facets, and use."

—Yogi Bhajan

Probably the most misunderstood type of yoga in the world is Tantric Yoga. It's really quite simple. There are three kinds of Tantric Yoga.

THREE TYPES OF TANTRIC

WHITE TANTRIC is to purify and uplift the being.

BLACK TANTRIC is for mental control of other people.

RED TANTRIC is for sexual energy and senses.

WHITE TANTRIC YOGA

Most energy we experience is either perpendicular or horizontal. Tantric energy is diagonal. White Tantric Yoga is the guided (by the Mahan Tantric) use of tantric energy which serves to accelerate the psychological transformation of the individual, dissolving deep-rooted subconscious neuroses. It is an ancient and very unique form of yogic science. It can only be practiced under the auspices and direction of the Mahan Tantric (Master of White Tantric Yoga), at a time and place specified by him.

You could search the world over, climb the highest mountains of Tibet, seek out the deepest caves of India and not find anyone else properly qualified to

179

teach you White Tantric Yoga, because the one and only person on the planet empowered to do so is Yogi Bhajan. He is the designated Mahan Tantric of this time.

Clearing out the deepest corridors of the subconscious mind, White Tantric Yoga is a very powerful group meditative experience. It uses mantra and yogic breathing techniques. You work with a partner. The Mahan Tantric connects with the students and guides the diagonal tantric energy using his subtle body. You can learn more about the subtle body in the chapter called "Ten Bodies."

White Tantric Yoga is not something that you can go home and practice on your own. This prohibition must be very strongly emphasized.

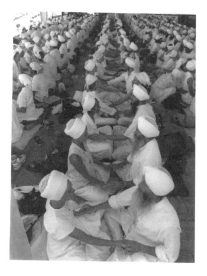

All the participants sit in rows, facing each other. The tantric energy travels in a zig-zag pattern up and down the rows. The students may meditate silently or at other times chant aloud, depending upon the instructions given. Sometimes the eyes are open, sometimes closed. Various mudras (hand positions) and postures are given. Although it is practiced with a partner, White Tantric Yoga is not a "sexual" yoga. On the contrary, it transmutes the sex energy from the lower chakras (energy centers) to the higher chakras.

In just a few minutes of White Tantric Yoga meditation you can accomplish results that would take months to achieve with any other practice. Yogi Bhajan says, "White Tantra is not the car, but it is taking the car through the car wash. Wax and clean and polish it, then keep it going."

Each person's experience of White Tantric Yoga is different. Each gets what he or she needs at that point in their journey along the path. It is a very deep and transformational cleansing process, yet people with no prior training or practice in yoga can participate in the Courses.

"From our childhood we have subconscious blocks and White Tantric Yoga is nothing but a conscious penetration through those blocks...It will give you a new start and a better life. It is neither a religion nor a philosophy, nor an exercise, nothing. It just works right there, in a couple of hours."[1]

We use the telephone to connect with other people at a distance, and we don't think that's unusual. The way we connect with the Mahan Tantric is very similar. We connect with him through his subtle body. He uses it to guide the diagonal tantric energy which penetrates and breaks up the blocks of anger, guilt, and fear buried in our subconscious. The Mahan Tantric does not have to be physically present to do his job. He has created Video courses in which he teaches White Tantric Yoga. He has given the privilege of facilitating these courses to a few individuals who travel with his video tapes on specific dates to specific cities. I hope you will have the opportunity to attend a White Tantric Yoga Course. There is nothing like it anywhere.

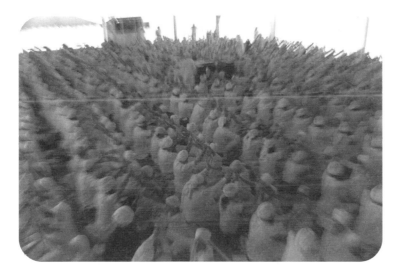

Just remember, in spirit, in flesh,
in eons, from time to time,
space to space, for centuries,
for lives we have been together,
playing the play of God
in the planet Earth, the Universe,
which is for us called life.
Sat Nam.
—*Yogi Bhajan, 1991*

25
The Ten Bodies

We know that we have a physical body. We can see it, touch it, feel it and so can other people (if we let them). But most of us are not aware that we have other bodies, which are equally real, if not more so. The funny thing is that we identify so strongly with our physical bodies, that we think of ourselves primarily in physical terms. It seems as if the physical body becomes the focus of our whole identity. As important and valuable as the physical body is, it is not who we are, because who we are, our essential self, can never change. You certainly don't have the same physical body you were born with, yet you know you're still you. Since this is practically the whole point of this book, I'm going to keep repeating it over and over: "you" are not your body or your mind(s). You are much more permanent than that. Sat Nam isn't born weighing six pounds-nine ounces, growing to 120 pounds; Sat Nam doesn't get the measles, go through menopause, or worry about dry skin. Sat Nam is your eternal true identity. It is who you are, who you were, and who you will be, now and forever. Truth is your identity.

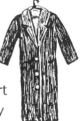

You might visualize your various bodies as layers of clothing, the physical body being the overcoat you wear for a lifetime. During your whole life, rain or shine, summer or winter, you never take it off, so you don't see the beautiful jacket or suit underneath, much less the dress or shirt under that. Until you develop a special kind of "x-ray" vision, you definitely never see the body that is wearing all those garments, which is the:

1. SOUL BODY

The first body is the Soul Body. It is your very best friend. It is God's light which lives in your heart. The Soul Body never dies. It goes with you forever. It's a good idea to get acquainted with it as soon as possible and develop an ongoing communication. Best time to get the conversation going is during morning sadhana. (See the chapter *Sadhana: Your Spiritual Bank Account* for a detailed guide to sadhana.)

2. THREE MENTAL BODIES

Here's a brief summary of the three main aspects of the Mind, the body that many people mistakenly identify with. You can read more about your mind(s) in the chapter called *Conquer the Mind, You Conquer the World*.

A. **THE NEGATIVE MIND** protects you by warning you what could be the danger or loss in any situation.

B. **THE POSITIVE MIND** inspires you by telling you what is the possible gain, the advantage to you, in any situation.

C. **THE NEUTRAL MIND** listens to the intellectual input from both the Negative Mind and the Positive Mind and then leads you to the best decision, using unbiased intuitive knowledge. Whenever you want to reach outside of yourself, reach out with your Neutral Mind. It is a most graceful, wonderful secret of success.

5. PHYSICAL BODY

The Physical Body was given to you so you could participate fully in life on this planet. It is a temple for God to live in while He sees through your eyes and hears through your ears. You were given the physical body so God could experience and enjoy (!) His creation. The physical is a balance point between heaven and earth. The key to perfecting the Physical Body is balance: balance in diet; balance in exercise; balance in work, in play, and rest. It always makes sense to avoid extremes. Don't be lazy and don't be fanatic.

6. PRANIC BODY

The Pranic Body controls the breath and takes in Prana, the life force energy of the universe. The Pranic Body gives you energy, courage, control over your mind, and healing power. When you breathe, you are feeding your Pranic Body. As you practice pranayam, you'll experience the expansion and strength of this body.

7. ARC BODY

The Arc Body is a line of energy that goes in an arc from ear tip to ear tip. It is sometimes called your "halo." This spiritual body projects who you are to other people without a word being spoken. It also protects you from negative energy directed towards you. Have you ever felt something, and turned around to find someone was staring at you? That's one experience of your arcline in action.

8. AURIC BODY

The Auric Body is a sphere of electromagnetic energy that surrounds the physical body. It can extend up to nine feet in every direction. This body protects you and also gives you the ability to uplift yourself and others. Some people can see the auric body as a field of flowing colored light. You may have experienced the auric body when you were near someone and simply felt their energy. Being in the aura of a spiritual and loving person is peaceful and healing. As the energy field of their aura interacts with ours, it automatically elevates us. (Remember, "Spirituality cannot be taught, It has to be caught, like the measles.You get it from someone who's got it.")

9. SUBTLE BODY

The Subtle Body gives you the opportunity to understand and master the subtlety of life. It can help you understand what is going on around you and how things work. Those people who can tune into situations easily or pick up new skills as if by magic, have developed the Subtle Body.

As the Mahan Tantric, Yogi Bhajan has explained that he always teaches with his Subtle Body. We have experienced the projection of his powerful presence during his White Tantric Yoga video courses. Even though his physical body may not be there, his Subtle Body most definitely is present and actively engaged with us.

10. RADIANT BODY

The Radiant Body gives you spiritual royalty and radiance. The strength of the Radiant Body will make you courageous in the face of any and every obstacle. Good things are drawn to you through a developed and powerful Radiant Body. On a practical level, people with well developed Radiant Bodies are said to have "charisma." Their very presence works for them before they say one word. They virtually "shine."

YOGI BHAJAN ON THE TEN BODIES

"You are a total combination of ten bodies. You have a Spiritual Body, you have three Mental Bodies (Negative, Positive, and Neutral); then you have this Physical Body, the Arc Body (which you call "halo"); and you have the simple Auric Body and a Subtle Body, Pranic Body, and a Radiant Body. These ten bodies are interlocked, but two are free to leave."

WHAT IS DEATH?

"Whenever the soul desires to leave the Physical Body, the Arc Body and all the other bodies remain behind because they have no combination. The Physical Body's pranic connection with the Pranic Body totally breaks, and the Soul leaves with the Subtle Body. That means, your identity is gone. (Your physical body remains, but "you" are gone. We call it death.)

"But do you understand what that indicates? If in subtlety you become very refined, and in activity you become very subtle, very subtle, you are very near to your Soul. The Spirit and the Subtle body are very much related. There's a direct relationship between the Subtle body and the Spiritual body. They never leave each other. So, anything you do which is refined — refined art, refined acts, refined speech, anything which is not gross — will put you nearer to the Soul. That's rather a simple way of reaching your God-consciousness."

26
Going Home

Yogi Bhajan Speaks on Death And Dying[1]

"What is death? Death is a process where your consciousness does not exist within the control of your ego. You can be brain-dead and still alive. Death — you share it every day with yourself. At a certain moment when you sleep you do not know if you are a man or a woman, or a person, or who you are, or what your status is, and you are "gone." It is that complete sleep in absolutely a state of turiya *(deep, dreamless sleep—see chapter on Sleep)* which gives your body what it needs for the next day. If that sleep is taken away from you for twenty-six days, you will die automatically, there is no lethal injection required.

If you do not understand, go to those people who cannot sleep at night. Look at their life and their story. It is most miserable.

"I have died once in my life. And I'll tell you my personal experience about death..." Yogi Bhajan went on to describe in detail a trip he took to a holy temple in India which was at the top of a very high mountain. He says "It was a very painful journey." After a long and strenuous climb, he was so hot and tired, as he puts it, he "did the biggest blunder of my life." He drank a glass of ice-cold water. The shock of the ice water must have been too much, for he collapsed on the ground. His friends carried him inside and sent for a doctor. When the doctor arrived, he was declared dead!

"...When I woke up, I had a blanket over my face." Then he saw everybody running around in excitement and distress. According to their records, he had been dead for 45 minutes. The doctor had declared him dead. But Yogi Bhajan woke up and said, "Oh, I was dead?" They said, "Sir, yes you were."

"Now I'm not? I'm alive?"

"Yes Sir, you are alive."

I said, "You are a doctor here?"

He said, "Yes, I'm a doctor."

I said, "How did I die?"

He said, "We do not know, outside at the stall you fell unconscious. So you were brought here and I examined you, and there was no heartbeat and everything was over with. And then your friends were running around trying to contact your headquarters to report that you were dead and to find out what to do next."

So, I asked for them to come in and I looked at them and said "I'm fine." Here he goes on to describe more of what he experienced while he was dead:

"...After I fainted, it was like a cylindrical round, what you call 'lift' (elevator). You might all be afraid of dying, but dying is the most beautiful, wonderful experience. Once in a while as a Yogi I get to that experience. (He then scientifically described the stage of meditation that brings ecstacy.) We then get into something like that. It's a great experience. I was thinking, thinking, thinking, going down, as our lifts sometimes go down, and down, and down and

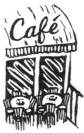

don't stop. And I came out. And there was a round square (like a town square). It was highly lit. There were two sides to it. Right and left. Left side like a bar or cafe. Very warm, very hot and people were talking, you could hear voices. And you see on that left side all your relatives. Believe me or not. And on the right side also you see relatives, but it is like a place with snow, like you are going to a hill station [Indian outposts high up in the mountains]. And you were right in the center, and from both sides your thought relatives call on you.

"I decided to come up. I took the lift, neither I went right nor I went left. I came back, sat in the lift, came up and I woke up and opened my eyes. That is my experience of death.

"And it shall happen to you all. What happens in death, when you have to die, you have exactly 30 seconds.

"There are three types of death. One is disease and sickness, you pay your karma and you struggle in the end of life. People say it's a miserable death. It's the best death because you take all the pain on your body. Martyrs take on their body, and humans take on their body and they pay their karma. It's a very painful death. It's every day, little by little, sickness. You know you are sinking, you know you are going and that's the last time when you can consciously connect with your infinity. You are going. Pain is there. HOW you are going, HOW you will deal with that pain.

HOW you can create conquering that pain ? If you can conquer that pain, in your

"Death is nothing but a good sleep."

language—not in my language—you have already found the "heavens." If you surrender to that pain, you have already found your hell. There's nothing in between. All this meditation, all this spirituality, all this whole getting up in the morning, three o'clock and cold water, two and a half hours, giving 1/10th of the earnings, having great temples made, and millions of people following you means nothing if you miss that 30 seconds. Period. All these practices are preparation towards death.

It doesn't mean a thing. It is absolutely a joke that all you do is to live. All your comforts are to live. You have never prepared to die. It amazes me - all over the world I go — that nobody understands this is the eventual un-defyable act. We all have to die. Whether you are a Sikh or a Hindu, Christian, you are short or tall, death is inevitable. And every day, meditatively you must die.

If you want no fear of death in the end, you have only one thing to do. You must voluntarily die. It's called turiya jagat suupanal...It's called turiya stage.'I can die, and I can live again,' consciously. And please find some good yogi, or a good teacher who can teach you. If you're a Jew, go to some Rabbi who knows about it. If you're Christian, find some Priest. If you're a Sikh...

"Death comes five times to every person. Four times it can be avoided, averted. Fifth time it happens.

"Death is nothing but a good sleep. A Sikh looks at death as union with the Beloved Creator. It is a time of joy because the soul has longed for this moment of utimate yoga (which means union). Sadness at this time is an experience of one's individual loss for the departed. Sikhs regard this time as an opportunity to love and accept God's will and sing His Praises."

YOU'RE HUMAN AREN'T YOU ?

Many years ago, I was devastated when a most wonderful young man, whom I loved very dearly, died in an automobile accident. Bhai Sahib Dayal Singh was barely twenty years old when he was killed. Despite my intellectual, philosophic acceptance of the fact that his death was surely a liberation for him, I was grief stricken. However, I believed I was supposed to maintain a stoic "yogic" non-attachment so I didn't want anyone, especially my spiritual teacher, to see me cry.

Yogi Bhajan had just returned from a lecture tour when he was told of Bhai Sahib Dayal Singh's death. There were several of us sitting in the living room, still in shock from the news. Every few minutes, overcome with emotion, I would go into the bathroom and cry. Then I would splash cold water on my face and return, trying to keep my composure. After a few such exits and entrances, Yogi Bhajan asked me what I was doing, I said, "I know I shouldn't cry, but..." He wouldn't let me finish the sentence. He simply said, "You're human aren't you?"

Yes, of course there is a legitimate reason and a need for grieving. It is to soothe and comfort us for our loss, for our feeling of separation, our missing the joy of that person being here with us. We go through a grieving process for our own well-being. Prayer, faith, and the loving support of friends and family can help us during a time of bereavement.

However, what the person who has died needs, is for us to let go, and release that soul, and not keep it tied to the earth with our grief. If we truly love someone, we will want to make their journey home to God smooth and direct.

There is a mantra to chant when someone dies. It sends out the vibrations that help carry a soul across all the planes to reach Home. That mantra is "AKAAL." Akaal means "undying." When someone has died, it is a Sikh practice for the congregation to chant AKAAL three to five times. The second syllable "kaal"—which means death—is held a long time. A deep breath precedes each repetition of the mantra. This is done during the Ardas, the traditional prayer, that is recited at every Sikh worship service and celebration. Anyone can use this mantra.

One of the most consoling experiences I have ever had was being able to help facilitate the transition when my mother died. She was 92, and had been seriously ill for some time. Even so, I found it hard to "let go." Cutting the umbilical cord at any age is more difficult than I had realized. By chanting AKAAL with four friends at her deathbed, I found myself greatly comforted and very grateful to know that I had done something to help her on her way.

Death is a fact of life. The more often we remind ourselves of the ultimate reality, that all things come from God and all things go to God eventually, including us, the easier it will be for us to handle that final journey home, for ourselves and for those whom we love.

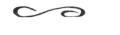

THE CHOICE

Two things are inevitable they say,
Death and taxes, you have to pay.

Country to country, taxes may vary
But death's a reality you simply can't bury.

It's only a body the soul is leaving behind
So, for a Yogi, it's liberation time!

Free at long last of the restrictions and limits
The physical body imposed
The Yogi, awake and aware, consciously chooses
The place where the soul finally goes.

There are two paths that open before you
When you leave earth plane below
One is warm and cozy, very appealing,
With friends and family that you know
Calling and beckoning, inviting you in
But it's a trap, delusion of maya trying to win
Trying to keep you from going beyond
And reaching your ultimate goal.
Turn away from temptation
Choose the road covered with the snow.

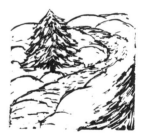

The cold and snowy route will take you Home where you belong
So when the time comes to turn left or right,
                    be sure to remember this song:

Take the cold and snowy route, ignore temptation please!
This final choice you have to make;
So you can meet your SELF, the GOD, with ease.

May the long time sun shine upon you
All love surround you
And the pure light within you
Guide your way on.

This "Sunshine Song[1]" is sung at the end of every 3HO event and every class in Kundalini Yoga. It is a positive affirmation bringing blessings to all.

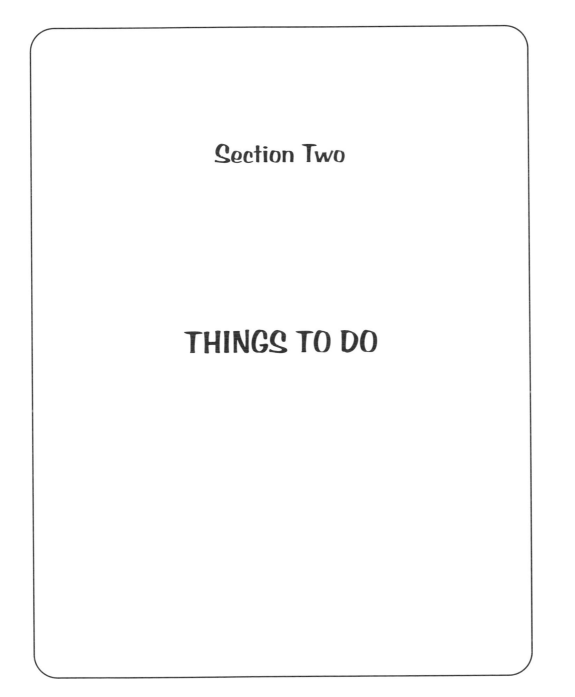

Section Two

THINGS TO DO

General Guidelines for the Practice of Kundalini Yoga

- Use common sense. If you have medical problems, consult with a doctor and let your Kundalini Yoga teacher know your situation.
- Begin each session by chanting **ONG NAMO GURU DEV NAMO**
- Breathe through your nose unless otherwise instructed.
- Wait at least one or preferably two hours after eating.
- Take your socks off. Best to have bare feet.
- Keep your spine covered.
- Ideally, stick to the prescribed times indicated in instructions. You may, however, *decrease* the time you do an exercise, if you need to, but do *not* increase the time that is specified.
- In general, it is advisable to relax briefly after each exercise, i.e., sit or lie down motionless, approximately 30 seconds to one minute.
- For maximum benefit anytime, unless another mantra is indicated, inhale thinking SAT and exhale thinking NAM.
- Ideally, cover your head.
- Women, please take special note: during the heaviest part of your monthly menstruation, avoid strenuous yoga. In particular do not do the following:

Bow Pose
Breath of Fire
Camel Pose
Locust Pose
Root Lock
Sat Kriya
Shoulder Stand or any inverted posture
Strenuous Leg Lifts

Mantra & Meditation

Key to Pronunciation

A	like the 'a' in about	OO	like the 'oo' in food
AA	like the 'a' in want	O	like the 'o' in go
AY	like the 'ay' in say	E	like the 'ay' in say
AI	like the 'a' in hand	EE	like the 'e' in meet
I	like the 'i' in bit	AAU	like the 'ow' in now
U	like the 'u' in put		

I must confess, some of the more common words that occur in the various mantras in this book have not been spelled according to the above key. For instance, the word "Guru" should probably be spelled G'roo,— but I don't like the way that looks, so I have to trust that you'll know how to pronounce it correctly wherever it appears! Similarly, "SAT NAM" would be spelled "Sat Naam" phonetically (though I have indicated near the beginning of the book that it rhymes with "but Mom"—unless you're from Canada where "mom" sounds like "mum"). Anyway, we'll try to catch all the places where you might need a clue to pronunciation, and spell phonetically for you. The best thing, of course, is to get a tape, or find a Kundalini Yoga teacher so you can listen and actually hear the sounds for yourself.

Beyond the above simple vowel sounds (I hope they're simple for you), some t's and d's, th's and dh's are reflexive, some are aspirated, but that's a bit more complicated than we need to deal with here. My suggestion is that if you're interested in a more detailed explanation of how to pronounce Gurumukhi (the language in which the sacred mantras were originally written) you read *Psyche of the Soul,* which does a wonderful job of explaining. You'll find it listed in the *Recommended Reading List* of books in the Sources and Resources section of this book.

How to Chant

The Technology
of Mantra

Here are some important guidelines to apply when chanting any mantra.

1. Remember, chanting is not singing or speaking, it is VIBRATING. You want to "feel" the mantra vibrating.

2. Keep your spine straight.

3. Chant from your navel point for maximum power.

4. HEAR the sound of the mantra coming through you. (After all, you aren't really chanting anyway, the One who breathes in you is doing it!)

5. If you're chanting with other people, listen to the leader and/or the group vibration and match it, stay with it.

6. When chanting aloud, be consciously aware of the activity of your tongue on the meridian points in the roof of your mouth. Some mantras, such as *Har,* or *Haree,* are supposed to be chanted only with the tip of the tongue, without moving the lips at all, while other mantras, such as *Wahe Guru*, at certain times, call for exaggerating the movement of the lips. Read all the instructions and follow them. Do the best you can, and let God do the rest!

WHY MEDITATE ?

"Meditation is one process through which you can resolve conflict and misfortune, rather than playing it through in real life. So for every child of a human, to learn the art of meditation is a must."[1]

- *Jap* is when you repeat with the tip of your tongue
- *Dhiaan* is when you meditate at the focal point at the tip of the nose or the chin with the optical nerve.[2]
- *Simran* is when you recite mentally.

203

"Man has two parts in the body which have to be worked on...That's the upper palate of the mouth and the frontal lobe of the forehead. If these two areas are undeveloped in your life, you don't have a chance. It doesn't matter despite all the education on this planet and everything else.

- Frontal lobe controls the personality.
- Upper palate, the hypothalamus, controls your automatic systems.

"You have to break the lead here (forehead). You have to meditate that way. That's why Kundalini Yoga is very easy and is for householders. It doesn't require any condition. It's just simple: Close your eyes nine-tenths, look at the tip of your nose. Or close your eyes, roll them down, look through the chin. And with the tip of the tongue, utter six words:

HAR HARAY HAREE WHA HE GURU

"Start practicing to develop your intuition. Lock your eyes at the tip of your nose and chant the mantra, "WA HE GURU." Your intuition will get clear in 90 days.

Sit with a straight spine. Close your eyes nine tenths of the way. Focus your eyes at the tip of the nose. Breathe long and deep. Listen to the tape, *Jai Ram, Siri Ram*[3]. After three minutes, inhale deep. Open your eyes. Relax.

"Whenever you will meditate like this,[4] this frontal lobe will become hard. And the more you meditate, it will become like lead. And the funny thing is, one day automatically it will not be lead. It's broken. You will have intuition to see the unseen, know the unknown, and hear the unheard. And your life will not be the same as you are now."[5]

Invoking the
Flow of Eternal Power

ONG NAMO GURU DEV NAMO

The first step in invoking the Flow Of Eternal Power in your life is to chant **Ong Namo Guru Dev Namo.** This mantra calls upon the Creator, the Divine Teacher, inside every human being. It establishes a strong and clear connection so that you can receive the highest guidance, energy, and inspiration. Always chant it before beginning any practice of Kundalini Yoga.

ONG is the Creator

NAMO means reverent greetings, salutations

GURU is the giver of the technology (GU= darkness, RU=light)

DEV means transparent (non-physical)

Ong Namo Guru Dev Namo is a very essential, important mantra.
Remember to chant it at least three times before you begin
each session of Kundalini Yoga.

(Detailed instructions for chanting are given in the chapter on Tuning In)

The Seed Sound

SAT NAM

SAT: Truth   NAM: Name, Identity

"Truth is your identity; God's Name is Truth."

SAT NAM (rhymes with "but mom"). It is the seed (bij) Mantra.
It reinforces the divine consciousness in everyone.
Use it as a greeting, anytime, anyplace.

By saying "Sat Nam" to each other, we acknowledge the highest consciousness in each of us. For that moment, we are relating as soul to soul, and we are truly "One in the spirit." (Then we can go on and agree or disagree about anything we want!)

➤ Linking the breath with **SAT NAM** is one of the easiest ways to maintain a constant reinforcement of your Self-awareness.
➤ Truth IS your identity.
➤ Inhale SAT and exhale NAM whenever you can.

**Wherever you go and whatever you do,
remember, SAT NAM lives and breathes in you.**

Raise the Kundalini

CHAKRA MEDITATION

In this meditation, you successively focus on each of the eight projected centers of consciousness, applying the Mul Bandh (Root Lock: *See Energy Up! in this section*) with each repetition of the mantra **SAT NAM**.

➤ Sitting in Easy Pose, spine straight, inhale deeply, chant **SAT NAM** (long drawn out syllable "Sat" and short "Nam" as you apply the Mul Bandh and concentrate at the **first chakra, the rectum**).

➤ Release the Root Lock, inhale deeply again, and chant **SAT NAM**, applying the Root Lock and focusing at the **second projected center of consciousness, the sex organ**.

➤ Release the Root Lock, inhale deeply, apply the Root Lock, chant **SAT NAM** as you focus on the **third center of consciousness, the navel point.**

➤ Continue this same process, going next to the **fourth chakra, the Heart Center**, at the center of the chest as you chant **SAT NAM** and apply the Root Lock.

➤ Then to the **Throat**, next to the **Third Eye** (between the eyebrows and up about 1/4 inch), then to the **top of the head** (the **Crown Chakra**) and with the eighth repetition of the mantra, visualize the sound going into the **Aura** that surrounds you.

You can repeat this complete sequence over and over again. Consciously bring your concentration successively up through all the chakras each time. Breathe very deeply before each repetition.

MEDITATION FOR CHANGE

SA-TA-NA-MA

31-Minute Meditation
The Power to Change Habit Patterns

Want to pull in all the loose ends, focus, and concentrate? Here's a mantra to help you consolidate and CHANGE YOUR HABITS. This mantra is a catalyst for change. So don't be surprised if your spiritual cleansing process is vastly accelerated! Be prepared, your status quo is about to be shifted into high gear.

Here's what the syllables mean:

SA	Totality (All that ever was, is or shall be)
TA	Creativity (The Principle of Creation)
NA	Destruction (Crucifixion)
MA	Regeneration (Resurrection)

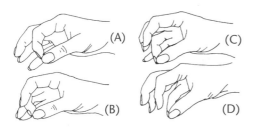

SA	thumb and forefinger (A)
TA	thumb and middle finger (B)
NA	thumb and ring finger (C)
MA	thumb and little finger (D)

Sit with your spine straight. Eyes are closed. With your hands resting on your knees, press the tip of the thumb of each hand firmly to each of the finger tips of that hand in sequence, starting with the forefingers while chanting each syllable in turn. Be sure as you chant each syllable to press firmly enough so that when you release the pressure, the tip of the finger is briefly white. If you press too gently you'll put yourself to sleep!

Keep moving your fingers throughout the entire meditation.

➤ First five minutes chant ALOUD
➤ Next five minutes chant in a LOUD WHISPER
➤ Eleven minutes chant SILENTLY
➤ Five minutes LOUD WHISPER
➤ Five minutes ALOUD

Inhale deeply, lift arms straight up in the air, vigorously shake out the fingers (approximately 1 minute). Relax.

SA TA NA MA is sometimes called the panch shabd (five sound current mantra). The fifth syllable is "A" which is common to the other four.

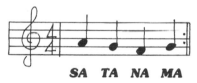

SA   TA   NA   MA

PICTURE THIS!
Meditation With Visualization

Although you do not have to know the meaning of the syllables, you may want to think about the concepts as you chant them. In fact, at one time Yogi Bhajan gave us some visual images to use while chanting this mantra. For those of you who would enjoy VISUALIZING, this is what he taught:

➤ Each time you chant "SA" picture all the galaxies, planets, suns, moons, and stars.
➤ Each time you chant "TA" visualize tremendous radiance, the brilliant, dazzling light of a trillion suns.
➤ Each time you chant "NA" see a winter landscape. The branches of the barren trees standing silent in the snow, all of nature dormant.
➤ Each time you chant "MA" picture thousands of spring flowers in a burst of glorious technicolor, brilliant blooms joyfully blanketing the hillside as far as the eye can see!

209

Change of Habit

Breath Meditation

The law of the universe is change. Everything changes. However, with every change in our life, one thing seems not to change: the attachment to our own ego. You can change, but your ego does not let you see your own maturity or potential. This creates a condition of constant hassle in the mind. The difference between your reality and your perception of it, through the ego, creates doubts and doubts create misery. Doubt steals three feet of your auric radiance. But the ego will not let you change easily. It blocks communication. You must assess yourself to come out of the darkness.

Ultimately, to be happy through all change and to have the full radiance of your soul, there must be surrender of your self to your higher Self. To aid the process of self-evaluation and to probe the ego to change and unblock subconscious communication, practice this meditation each day.[1]

Sit with a very straight spine. Lift the chest. Curl the fingers in, as if making a fist. The finger tips will be on the pads of the hands. Then bring the two hands together at the center of the chest. The hands will touch lightly in two places only: the knuckles of the middle (Saturn) fingers and the pads of the thumbs. The thumbs are extended toward the heart center and are pressed together

Hold this position as you feel the energy across the thumbs and knuckles. Begin long, deep and full breathing. Concentrate on the flow of the breath. Continue for 31 minutes. Then inhale deeply and relax for 5 minutes. After practicing and mastering this time for the kriya, you can extend the time to do it for another 31 minutes after the rest period.

210

MANTRA OF PROTECTION

Aad Guray Nameh
Jugaad Guray Nameh
Sat Guray Nameh
Siri Guru Dayvay Nameh

ACCIDENTS

There's no such thing as an "accident." An accident is the result of time and space coordinates triggering an event. Accidents happen when you're in a certain place at a certain time. Maybe it's the right place at the wrong time or the wrong place at the right time!

Here's a yogic "secret" to enable you to protect yourself from accident and incident. It creates a cushion, a buffer of time, which changes your future location in space.

This mantra of protection gives you an edge over time and space. It only takes a few seconds to repeat it a couple of times before you turn the key in the ignition. Those few seconds create a margin of safe-

Accidents don't just happen, they are caused.

ty of about nine feet at that crucial moment in time when you might otherwise have met an accident. (Also, I wouldn't underestimate the power of the consciousness you are invoking with these particular syllables. See the following explanation.)

MANTRA OF PROTECTION

Protection and guidance are always with us. It is in our very core. Only we are blind to it at times. To clear the clouds and open ourselves to receive that guidance and protection we use this mantra. We call on the sources of wisdom and teaching that are within us.

Aad Guray Nameh

Jugaad Guray Nameh

Sat Guray Nameh

Siri Guru Dayvay Nameh

- **Nameh** is a reverent invocation, it opens the gates to the guidance.
- **Guray** means the knowledge or teaching itself.
- **Aad** is guidance at the beginning of each action or thought.
- **Jugaad** is guidance through time, both timeless and timely!
- **Sat** is guidance through every experience by remembering the true essence and purpose.
- **Siri** is that great guidance beyond what we know; it is the higher self answering questions we have not even asked.
- **Guru** is the giver of the technology (dispeller of ignorance).
- **Davay** means "transparent," i.e. non-physical.

All together, this protects you completely. You can recite it in a monotone or sing it to a melody, but USE IT!

MEDITATION FOR POSITIVE COMMUNICATION

"This meditation will give you the ability to get out of all negativity and always have the power to communicate positively."[1]

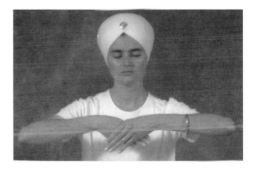

Sit in Easy Pose with a straight spine. Both palms face the body with the back of the right hand in the palm of the left. The fingers of both hands are straight. Fold the left thumb over the right palm and fold the right thumb over the left thumb. The hands will be crossed with the fingers angled downward. Lock the thumb in place. (If you are left-handed, reverse the hand position.) Hold arms at shoulder level parallel to the floor. Stretch the shoulders forward. The hands should be 9 to 12 inches from the chest.

Eyes are closed. The mantra is:

HAREE HAREE HAREE HAREE HAREE HAREE HAR

Deeply inhale through the nose, then chant the mantra five times in a monotone as you exhale. Be sure to use up all the breath as you chant. Then inhale and begin again. Continue for 3, 11, or 31 minutes.

This meditation and the one on the following page are for improving communication skills and were first published in "Communication: Liberation or Condemnation," Yogi Bhajan's Ph.D. Dissertation.

MEDITATION TO DEVELOP EFFECTIVE COMMUNICATION

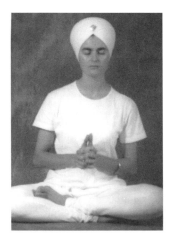

Sit in an easy cross-legged position with spine straight or in a chair with both feet on the ground with weight equally distributed between them. Interlock the fingers with the right index finger on top of the left index finger and the thumbs joined and pointing straight up. Hold the position in front of chest between the solar plexus and the heart. Relax the arms down with the elbows bent and the forearms pulled up and in toward the chest until the hands have met between the levels of the solar plexus and the heart. Eyes are closed. Inhale deeply through the nose and chant the mantra as you exhale completely.

Raa, Raa, Raa, Raa
Maa, Maa, Maa, Maa
Saa, Saa, Saa, Sat
Haree Har Haree Har

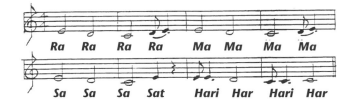

The word **"SAT"** rhymes with "but."

When you chant the line Haree Har Haree Har, do not move the lips; pronounce this line with the tongue, as if there were no vowel in the syllable "har".

Be sure to chant the entire mantra on each full exhalation.

Mentally focus on the breath and the chanted mantra.

There are no time restrictions. Practice this on an empty stomach.

This meditation will make your language very effective, so effective you will be able to communicate through the sheer force of your thoughts.

214

"LONG EK ONG KAR'S"
(My Favorite Mantra)

EK ONG KAR SAT NAM SIRI WAHE GURU
Two-and-a-Half Breath Cycle

Ek (One)

Ong (Creator)

Kar (Creation)

Sat (Truth)

Nam (Name)

Siri (Great)

Wahe (Beyond description—"wow!")

Guru (Dispeller of darkness, Divine Teacher within)

This mantra opens the chakras. These eight words are the "code" letters, or the phone number of the direct line to "connect" you, the creature, with your Creator. It was the first, and almost the only mantra Yogi Bhajan taught during his first year in the United States. I must admit, it's my favorite. When chanted powerfully, it is extremely energizing.

The ideal, most effective time of day to chant is during what are called the Ambrosial Hours, the two and one-half hours before sunrise in the morning. (Since 1992, 3HO students and teachers have been chanting "Long Ek Ong Kar's" for seven minutes to begin the one hour of chanting during morning sadhana. It is followed by six other mantras, making up a full hour of chanting.) On August 26th every year, we synchronize our clocks and chant the mantra *Guru Guru Wahe Guru Guru Ram Das Guru* for eleven minutes simultaneously all over the world (3 a.m. in Los Angeles, 6 a.m. in New York, etc.), followed or preceded by "Long Ek Ong Kar's" for two-and-a-half hours, to celebrate Yogi Bhajan's birthday.

It has been said that a person can attain liberation by chanting this mantra correctly, for two-and-a-half hours before sunrise for 40 days. (Correctly would mean with full concentration.)

Other suggested time periods for personal practice of this mantra are thirty-one minutes or one hour. The two essential requirements are:

1. Sit with a straight spine.
2. Apply the Neck Lock (pull chin straight back).

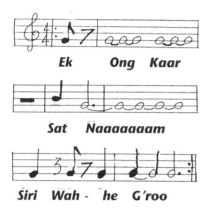

Ek   Ong   Kaar

Sat   Naaaaaaam

Siri Wah - he G'roo

Inhale deeply and chant **EK ONG KAR**

Inhale deeply again and chant **SAT Naaam** until you're almost out of breath, then REACH for the **S'ree**, which is brief. Then ...

Inhale 1/2 Breath and chant **WAH** - (hay) **G'roo**

Inhale deeply again to repeat the cycle.
Continue for 11 minutes, or longer.

Points to remember:

➤ **EK** is vibrated powerfully at the Navel Point (not shouted).

➤ **ONG** is chanted at the back of the throat, vibrates the upper palate and comes out through the nose. Slide into the KAR without a pause.

➤ **SAT** is powerfully chanted at the Navel point and NAAM seems to vibrate at the heart center.

➤ The **SIRI** is pronounced as if spelled S'REE — but it is a short syllable, and the **WAH** is also short and somewhat aspirated.

➤ **HE** (pronounced hay) is extremely short and briefly precedes the **GURU** which is pronounced "g'roo".

216

MEDITATION TO CLEAR
PAST, PRESENT, AND FUTURE

"When you cannot be protected, this mantra shall protect you. When things stop, and won't move, this makes them move in your direction."[1]

This mantra must be chanted aloud. But you can chant it any time, any place. Sitting, standing, walking, swimming, cooking, ironing, or even jumping out of an airplane: it doesn't matter what posture you're in, or what time of day it is!

CHANT ALOUD FOR EXACTLY 31 MINUTES EVERY DAY.
Ten minutes cover your past, ten are for the present, ten for the future, and one minute is for infinity.

Aad Guray Nameh
Jugaad Guray Nameh
Sat Guray Nameh
Siri Guru Dayvay Nameh

Aad Such Jugaad Such Haibhee Such
Nanak Hosee Bhee Such

Aad Such Jugaad Such Haibhay Such
Nanak Hosee Bhay Such

217

This meditation combines three separate mantras, each of which enjoys its own individual power and purpose. When chanted in this sequence, they become a formula to clear our karmic debts: past, present, and future!

• The first mantra of this three part meditation is a mantra of protection. *(Aad Guray Nameh... It has already been explained as the Mantra of Protection.)*

• The second mantra (..."bhee" such) is from Guru Nanak's *Japji Sahib.* *(Aad Such, Jugaad Such, Habhee Such, Nanak Hosee Bhee Such . Its literal meaning is:* True in the beginning, True through all the ages, True even now, Nanak says Truth shall always exist.)

• The third mantra has the same translation, but *"bhay" such* acts to remove obstacles. It was originally given to Guru Arjan Dev when he was composing *Sukhmani Sahib* and had writers block.

BE AWARE !

• Note the important difference in pronunciation between:

Haibee: The mantra using *"bhee"* acts as a generator,
and
Haibhay: The mantra using *"bhay"* acts as a lever.

• Be sure to really emphasize the "ch" sound at the end of every "such."

"MAY THE FORCE BE WITH YOU"

Yogi Bhajan says,

"Whoever recites this mantra becomes absolutely divine, God in action. Pavan is 'May the force be with you.' This mantra increases the pranic energy. There is no better healing than this."

PAVAN PAVAN PAVAN PAVAN
PAR PARAA PAVAN GURU
PAVAN GURU WAHE GURU
WAHE GURU PAVAN GURU

"Pavan" means the carrier of the "prana," the life force.

Pronounce the consonant "v" very softly, almost like a "w" and "roll" the "r"s slightly. *(See Pronunciation Guide)*

Musical Tape #GSK007, Guru Shabad Singh Khalsa, Golden Temple Recordings

Shout it in the Shower!

ANG SANG WAHE GURU

A sure-fire time to remember God is when you step into your shower first thing in the morning. When that cold water hits you *(Yes, cold, remember it's hydrothermal therapy explained in the How to Get Up in the Morning chapter!)*, instead of shrieking "Oh my God!" (which at least has you thinking in the right direction) you might try shouting **ANG SANG WAHE GURU!** *(Pronounced "ung sung waa(hay) g'roo.")*

Any time is a good time to use this mantra. It is recommended to repeat it at least 26 times every day of your life.

ANG SANG WAHE GURU means "God is in every part of me." Every limb, every joint. In other words,

GOD AND ME, ME AND GOD ARE ONE

This may not be the best grammar, but it's a statement of Truth. And truth carries power. The more you think of yourself as a Divine Being, the easier it is for that reality to manifest. Use these words as a positive affirmation to awaken your soul.

THE PERSIAN WHEEL

(Gatga)

*When your smile disappears and you wear a frown
It shows your thinking's upside down.*

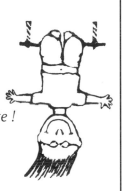

*Better look at your mind and see what's in it—
then with this mantra, you can fix it in a minute !*

*Whatever the worry that's pulling you down
You can use this sound to turn it around*

*EK ONG KAR SAT GUR PRASAAD,
SAT GUR PRASAAD EK ONG KAR*

*It's quite simple, why not try it,
Give it a whirl, I think you'll buy it !*

*Repeat five times, it will change your mood
from negative to positive —
From rotten —-feel good !*

*Like the tiny stick on the Persian wheel
That works to reverse the spin
This mantra controls the mind
No matter what state you're in*

*Change your direction and you will see
From mind's domination you'll be free.*

221

Kriyas & Pranayam

Exercises & Breathing

Energy Up!
Mul Bandh (Root Lock)

This lock is the most frequently used in the practice of Kundalini Yoga. It closes off the three lower chakras and allows the Kundalini energy to rise. Try this:

Sit in easy pose. Inhale deeply, as deeply as you can, and exhale, still holding the chest high. With the breath held out, simultaneously contract (squeeze) the muscles of the rectum, the sex organ, and the navel point — pulling in and up on the navel. Inhale, relax the contraction, exhale, and repeat. Practice this for several minutes. Mul Bandh can be applied with breath held in or out; the breath will be specified in the exercise given.

SAT KRIYA

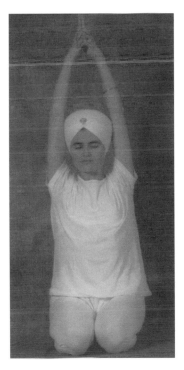

Now that you know how to apply the root lock, you can use it to experience one of the most powerful kriyas in all of the Kundalini technology. If there were only one kriya that I could share with you, this is the one I would choose.

Sitting on your heels, place your arms over your head, palms together, interlacing your fingers, index fingers pointing up. Your upper arms are hugging your ears. Keep the arms straight, do not bend the elbows.

There is no special breathing specified for Sat Kriya, because the breath will take care of itself. There is no retention while you're chanting, only at the very end of the kriya, you'll hold the breath in or out, as directed.

Close your eyes. Keep them closed and focus them at your third eye point (between the eyebrows and up slightly, about one-quarter to one-half inch). Maintain this focus throughout the exercise.

Inhale slightly to begin, and powerfully chant aloud the syllable **SAT**. (SAT NAM rhymes with "but mom.") vibrating it from your navel point as you apply the Root Lock. If you pull in and up strongly enough on the navel, and your arms are reaching up high enough, the Mul Bandh will almost automatically be applied. The sound should be very powerful, but not necessarily loud. It does not have to be shouted. The power of it can be felt, as a vibration. Then release the Root Lock as you chant the word **NAAM**.

NAAM is short, the syllable is not extended. It may be barely audible. Continue chanting SAT NAM as you contract the muscles of the rectum and sex organ, pulling in and up simultaneously on the navel point each time you chant the syllable SAT. Beginners, continue only for forty-five seconds to one minute.

Inhale deeply and with the breath held in, apply the Root Lock tightly as you squeeze the energy up from the base of the spine to the top of the skull. Hold about five to ten seconds. Exhale, and inhale again, repeat the Root Lock and squeeze the energy up. Third time, inhale deeply and this time exhale completely out and holding the breath out, apply the Root Lock, squeezing the energy all the way up, up, up and out the top of your head — hold for a maximum of eight seconds. Inhale, exhale and sweep your arms out to the sides and down in an arc. Relax and sit very still with your eyes closed for at least one minute, meditating at the third eye point.

"KEEP UP and you'll be kept up."

—Yogi Bhajan

As you practice this kriya daily, you can gradually increase the time to three minutes. Eventually, Sat Kriya can be done for as long as thirty-one minutes, but you must work up to this gradually.

It has been said that the period of relaxation after Sat Kriya should be equal in length to the time of the kriya.

Sat Kriya will raise your kundalini. Then it is up to you to "Keep Up!"

Sharpen Your Mind

Basic Breath Series[1]

Find a quiet spot, where you won't be disturbed and you won't be conspicuous! You can do this sitting in a chair if you can't sit on the floor. Just make sure your spine is straight and you're not going to fall. Both feet should be flat on the floor with weight equally distributed. This is a Pranayam to make the mind sharp and clear, and able to focus on many things. (As you practice this breathing sequence, you can be linking your breath with a mantra, using your mind to hear the sound **SAT** on the inhale and **NAAM** on the exhale.)

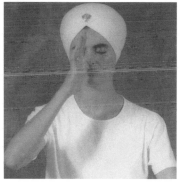

1) Sitting in Easy Pose. Close off your right nostril with your right thumb and breathe long and deep through your left nostril for 3 minutes.

2) Change hands and close off the left nostril. Breathe slowly and deeply through the right nostril only, for 3 minutes.

3) Repeat breath through left nostril only, 1 minute.

4) Repeat breath through right nostril only, 1 minute.

5) Using thumb and little finger, close alternate nostrils so that you inhale through the left and exhale through the right (1-3 minutes).

6) Reverse the sequence and inhale through the right and exhale through the left (1-3 minutes).

7) Inhale through both nostrils and begin Breath of Fire for 3 minutes. (You can build up time to 7 minutes as optimum.)

8) Relax or meditate for 5 minutes.

9) Chant long "Sat Nam's."

This is an excellent pranayam to do as preparation for a set of Kundalini Yoga exercises, or any strenuous activity.

Loosen Up/Tune Up
Kriya For Elevation

"You may die, but you'll never grow old if you have a flexible spine."
—Yogi Bhajan

You've heard the expression "Loosen up!" or "Don't be up-tight!" It's good advice. We need a flexible spine to make our attitude flexible, to be able to relax and yet be strong. When the spine is rigid, the energy can't flow freely. Did you ever notice that age and rigidity seem to go together? If we want to feel "young" (i.e., active, enthusiastic, energetic) at any age, we need flexibility. Physically, it starts with the spine.

The 72,000 nerves in the body draw energy from the twenty-six vertebrae in the spine. In the spine are control centers, and if there is tension or blockage in the spine, you can't have a correct perspective on life.

Here's a set of exercises to help make your spine flexible and strengthen those important nerve centers in the spine, plus much more.

KRIYA FOR ELEVATION
as taught by Yogi Bhajan, Master of Kundalini Yoga

What does it do?
- This Kriya is a good warm up and tune up
- Systematically exercises the spine
- Aids in circulation of Prana to balance the Chakras

Remember to think **SAT** as you inhale, **NAAM** as you exhale, to increase the power and elevate your consciousness with every exercise.

KRIYA FOR ELEVATION

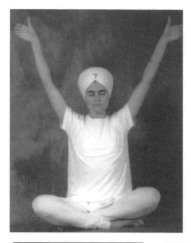

1. This exercise is sometimes called the **Ego Buster.** Sit in Easy Pose. Bring your arms up at a 60 degree angle out to the sides. Curl your fingertips onto the pads at the top of the palms, just before the fingers begin. Thumbs point straight up. Breath of Fire 1 to 3 minutes. Keep your arms straight; no bend in the elbows. Stretch up from your arm pits.

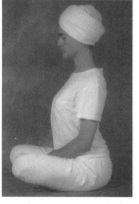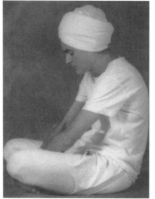

2. **Camel Ride**. Sitting in Easy Pose, hold on to your shins with your hands and flex your spine. Inhale as you lift the chest up high, pulling in the lower back; exhale as you relax the spine out, drop the chest, and droop the shoulders forward. It is a continuous fluid motion. Continue with a powerful breath: 1 to 3 minutes. Think of your spine as a wet noodle or a rubber band. Use your arms to pull your spine gently forward each time you inhale.

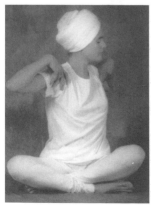

3. **Spinal Twist**. Sitting in Easy Pose, put your hands on your shoulders, thumbs behind, fingers in front. Inhale as you twist to the left and exhale as you twist to the right. The head moves with the body. Twist, 1 to 3 minutes.

KRIYA FOR ELEVATION

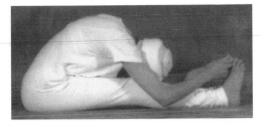

4. **Life nerve stretch**. Sit with your legs stretched out in front. Grab the big toe of each foot. (Socks are off.) Lock each index finger around the big toe and press the thumb against the nail while applying pressure to the ball of the toe. Keeping the backs of the knees flat on the floor, inhale and sit up, stretching the spine straight, pulling back on toes. Exhale, bend forward, pulling elbows to the ground, head to knees. Continue with deep powerful breath 1 to 3 minutes. Do the best you can, even if you're only bending a centimeter in each direction! The object of this exercise is to stretch the nerve that runs up the back of the leg behind the knee and develop flexibility of the spine. It will loosen up with practice.

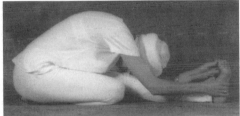

5. Sit on your right heel with your left leg extended forward. Grasp the big toe of the left foot with your left hand and hold on to the instep with your right hand. Bend your head to your knee (if you can). Breath of Fire 1 to 2 minutes. Inhale, Exhale, and stretch forward and down, hold the breath out briefly. Then Inhale, switch legs, and repeat with Breath of Fire for 1 minute. Switch legs and repeat for 30 seconds on each leg. This exercise helps to get the toxins out of the system. Breathe powerfully.

6. Sit with your legs spread wide apart. Grab on to your toes, keeping the backs of your knees flat on the ground. Inhale and stretch your spine straight up as much as you can, holding on to the toes. Exhale, bend at the waist, bringing your head down toward the right knee. Inhale straight up to the center, exhale down to the left. If you can't reach all the way to your toes, hold onto the calves of the legs or wherever you can reach without bending the knees. Continue 1 to 2 minutes breathing powerfully. To end the exercise, exhale, stretch forward, and hold the breath out briefly. Then inhale up and relax. This exercise charges the magnetic field.

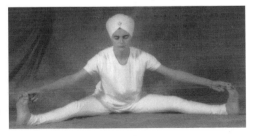

231

KRIYA FOR ELEVATION

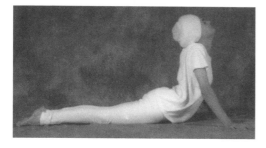

7. **Cobra Pose**. Lie on your stomach with the palms flat on the floor under your shoulders, fingers facing forward. The heels are together with the soles of the feet facing up. Inhale into Cobra Pose, arching your spine vertebra by vertebra from the neck to the base of the spine until the arms are straight with the elbows locked. Begin Breath of Fire. Continue for 1 to 3 minutes. Then inhale, arching the spine to the maximum. Exhale and hold the breath out briefly, apply the Root Lock (Mul bandh). Inhale deeply, then exhaling, slowly lower the arms and relax the spine, vertebra by vertebra from the base of the spine to the top. Relax, lying on your stomach with the chin on the floor and the arms by the sides. This exercise balances the sexual energy and draws the prana to balance apana so that the kundalini energy can circulate to the higher centers in the following exercises.

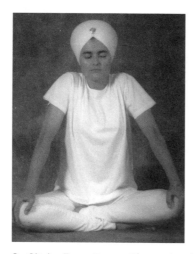

8. Sit in Easy Pose. Place the hands on the knees. Inhale and shrug your shoulders as high as you can up toward your ears. Exhale and drop the shoulders down. Continue rhythmically with powerful breathing for 1 or 2 minutes. Inhale. Exhale and relax. This exercise balances the upper chakras and opens the hormonal gate to the higher brain centers.

9. Sit in Easy Pose. Begin rolling the neck clockwise in a circular motion, bringing the right ear toward the right shoulder, the back of the head toward the back of the neck, the left ear toward the left shoulder and the chin toward the chest. The shoulders remain relaxed and motionless, and the neck should be allowed to gently stretch as the head circles around. Continue for 1 or 2 minutes, then reverse the direction and continue for 1 or 2 minutes more. Bring the head to a central position and relax.

232

KRIYA FOR ELEVATION

10. **Sat Kriya**. Sit on your heels in the Sat Kriya position. Stretch your arms over your head so that the upper arms are hugging your ears. Interlace your fingers except for the index fingers which are pressed together and pointing up. Begin to chant "SAT NAM" emphatically in a constant rhythm about 8 times per 10 seconds. (Don't speed up.) Chant the sound "SAT" from the navel point and solar plexus, and pull the navel all the way in toward the spine as you apply the Root Lock. On "NAM" relax the lock. Continue for 3 to 7 minutes, then inhale and squeeze the muscles tight from the buttocks all the way up the back past the shoulders. Mentally allow the energy to flow through the top of the skull. Exhale. Inhale deeply. Exhale completely and apply the Mul Bandh with the breath held out. Inhale and relax. Sat Kriya circulates the kundalini energy through the cycle of the chakras, aids in digestion, and strengthens the nervous system.

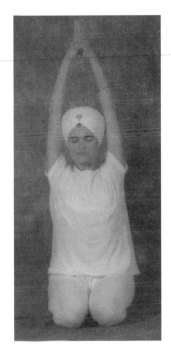

11. Relax in Easy Pose or on your back with the arms at the sides, palms up. Deep relaxation allows you to enjoy and consciously integrate the mind\body changes which have been brought about during the practice of this kriya. It allows you to sense the extension of the self through the magnetic field and the aura and allows the physical body to deeply relax.

This "Kriya for Elevation" was printed in the yoga manual "Keeping Up with Kundalini Yoga." It can be done in 20 minutes or take as long as 50 minutes, depending upon how long you continue each exercise. Time options are listed.

Reprinted by permission.

233

Easy Set

I call this the "Easy Set," because four out of the five exercises are done lying down! It is one of the earliest sets Yogi Bhajan taught in Los Angeles (February 13, 1969). A Valentine's Day gift perhaps?

Breathe very powerfully as you do the exercises so that you can

➤ Increase your lung capacity,

➤ Eliminate toxins from your system,

➤ Make your "beauty gland" secrete,

➤ Work on your eyesight.

1. INCREASE YOUR LUNG CAPACITY.

Lie on your back, interlace your fingers in a loose Venus Lock at the back of your neck. Be sure your fingers are underneath your hair.

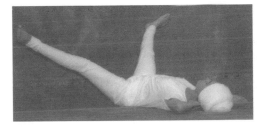

   a) Legs are spread apart 3 feet. Breath of Fire 2 to 3 minutes.

   b) Inhale and keeping the legs apart raise them up to a 60 degree angle, hold the breath, and keep the legs up for 20 seconds.

   Exhale and s-l-o-w-l-y lower the legs down (still spread apart). Take at least 10 seconds to lower.

   c) Repeat (b).

   d) Relax.

EASY SET

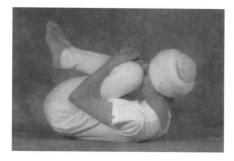

2. **ELIMINATE TOXINS.** Lying on your back, press your knees tightly against your lungs, holding them in place with your hands locked around them. Raise your head and bring your nose right into the knees. Breath of Fire 30 seconds to 1 minute. This is working with the "apana vayu," the eliminating force which takes away everything not required by the body. Relax.

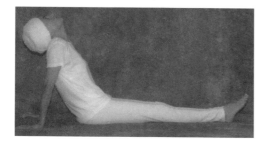

3. **MAKE YOUR THYROID SECRETE.** The Thyroid relates to your skin, complexion, outward appearance, and energy level. Sit up. Lean back 60 degrees. Brace yourself with your arms behind you. Look at the ceiling, don't wink. Fix your eyesight at one point. Breath of Fire for 1 to 2 minutes. Don't blink, let your eyes water. Inhale. Hold briefly, exhale, relax. This exercise also works on headaches and eyesight.

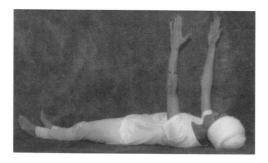

4. Lying on your back, inhale deeply and raise your hands to the ceiling, stretching your arms up from your shoulders. Extend the fingers out as if reaching for a star, then,

236

holding the breath, slowly and powerfully bend your fingers to make the hands into fists and bending your elbows, bring the fists s-l-o-w-l-y down to your chest, as if you are fighting a resistance to that movement. Your arms will shake. Exhale when your fists touch your chest. Inhale and repeat the exercise.

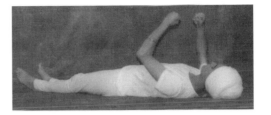

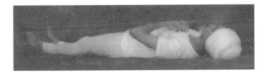

5. Lying on your back, arms at your sides. Breath of Fire for 1 minute.

   Inhale, and keeping your feet flat on the ground, raise your waistline up, making an arc of the body. Hold briefly, and exhale down.

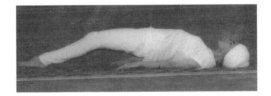

6. Relax completely in Corpse Pose.

Balance Your Glands
What's Your Angle?

Glands are the guardians of your health.

One of the main reasons why Kundalini Yoga works so fast and effectively is its use of angles. This is one of the "secrets" of its success.

Lifting the legs to different heights creates pressure on specific glands and organs depending upon the angle of the lift. Pressuring the glands causes them to secrete. When the pressure is released, and the body is held motionless, the glandular secretions that have been stimulated have an opportunity to circulate freely throughout the body. The result is a balanced glandular system.

In addition to your nervous system, your glandular balance has a definite effect on your emotional stability through the chemistry of your body. Glands are the guardians of your health. Your glandular fluctuations can make you feel depressed or elated. Glandular changes cause mood swings. So a medical check-up is not a bad idea. However, we should mention that in India, when the doctors have done everything they can for a patient, and they don't know what else to do, they send them to the yogis!

In the Orient, yogic therapists are acknowledged and respected as specialists in nerves, glands, and natural methods of self-healing, including diet.

We're not doctors and we don't make any medical claims, but we have seen that the practice of Kundalini Yoga results in improving physical health, mental clarity, and emotional balance and control.

WHAT DO THE GLANDS DO?

Here's a quick highlighting of the tasks a few of our glands perform for us:

PANCREAS

The pancreas' job is to keep the blood-sugar level in the bloodstream constant. It is very important in the digestive process and must secrete an adequate supply of the insulin hormone, otherwise diabetes results. Overworking the pancreas (by overloading it with excessive carbohydrates, as I did during a time in my life when I was eating three candy bars a day) can cause a condition known as hypoglycemia in which the pancreas can't do its job properly and a person can suffer severe mood swings, among other symptoms.[1]

THE TWO DIVINE GLANDS
Pituitary

The pineal and pituitary glands are known by the yogis as the "divine glands" because they are so closely connected with our higher states of consciousness. The pituitary is the master gland of the body; it controls other endocrine glands and affects growth, memory functions, and intuition.

Pineal

Although modern science has finally discovered that the pineal gland affects all the rhythms of our activity, the full functions of the pineal are not yet documented in the West.

TWO BEAUTY GLANDS: Thyroid and Parathyroid

These are known as the "beauty" glands. Your energy level is affected by the thyroid. Underactive secretion of the thyroid can make you feel depressed and lethargic. The thyroid hormone increases the rate of oxidation in the body (producing heat) and of sugar metabolism. It also promotes growth, ossification of bones, and development of teeth, plus it stimulates the nervous system, the adrenals, and the gonads.

240

The parathyroid hormone regulates the metabolism of bones and maintains normal functioning of the nerves and the muscles, including the heart.

GEOMETRY THEY DIDN'T TEACH IN SCHOOL

Here's what happens when the legs are lifted to various heights doing Kundalini Yoga :

➤ 0 to 12 inches affects everything below the navel point: the creative glands, sex organs, ovaries, uterus, digestive glands, intestines, and eliminating glands.

➤ 0 to 6 inches: specifically affects ovaries/sex glands

➤ 6 to 18 inches: navel point, kidneys

➤ 12 inches to 2 feet: liver, spleen, gall bladder, pancreas

➤ 1 1/2 feet to 2 1/2 feet : liver, upper stomach, gall bladder

➤ 2 to 3 feet: heart, lungs, stomach

➤ Over 4 feet to 90°: thyroid, parathyroid, pineal

➤ 90°: memory, control centers (pineal and pituitary)

ANGLES

as taught by Yogi Bhajan—1969

Here's a set of exercises that is a little more strenuous than some of the other beginners' sets. Yogi Bhajan gave it during the first year he taught in America, when we were all beginners. It works on strengthening the energy field of the body and balancing the glandular system. Try it. See how well you can do. Remember, Kundalini Yoga is not a competitive sport. The only person you have to challenge is yourself, to see how quickly you can build your endurance and stamina.

Truly, the difference between practicing a set of exercises as a beginner or as an advanced student is usually the ability to "keep up" for the entire time specified. If an exercise calls for three minutes, a beginner may be able to do it only for one minute, and that's okay! Times listed are the ideal, but they are also the maximum. Even if you are an advanced student, do NOT go beyond the time specified.

241

WHAT'S YOUR ANGLE?

HERE'S WHAT TO DO

Sit with a straight spine. Remember to breathe only through your nose. You will be using alternate nostrils to inhale and exhale. You can use the thumb and little finger of one hand to close off the alternate nostrils.

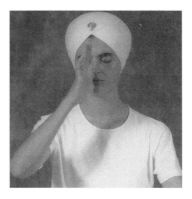

1. First, close off your right nostril and inhale deeply through the left nostril. Immediately close off the left nostril and exhale through the right. Continue. Take ten long deep breaths, inhaling through the left, exhaling through the right. Make each inhalation and each exhalation as long and deep as you possibly can. This way of breathing deals with the electric field of the body, and helps balance the two hemispheres of the brain.

2. Lie on your back, raise your legs 6 inches from the ground and begin scissoring them (criss-crossing), keeping them at the 6-inch height parallel to the ground. This sends energy to the brain cells. (The yogis claimed it also bestowed longevity.) 1 to 3 minutes. Relax at least 1 minute.

WHAT'S YOUR ANGLE?

3. Raise your left leg up 12 inches as you inhale; exhale and lower it. Inhale and raise your right leg up 12 inches; exhale and lower it. Consciously use your breath to lift each leg. Continue lifting your legs alternately to a height of 12

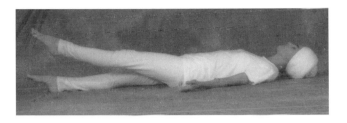

inches, breathing deeply through both nostrils. This exercise affects the creative glands. Continue at a moderate pace for 2 to 5 minutes, then immediately inhale deeply and raise both feet at the same time to a 6 inch height. Hold steady for a few seconds with the breath held in. Exhale, slowly lowering the legs. Repeat these double leg lifts for a total of three times. Relax.

4. Still lying on your back, bring your arms up and overhead behind you on the floor. Keeping the arms next to your head, inhale and sit up, exhale and bend forward to touch your toes, inhale sit up again, exhale, lie back down. Repeat five times.

5. Lie in corpse pose and relax completely for five to ten minutes. (Flat on your back, with your arms at your sides, palms up. Keep your body in a straight line.)

Two things to avoid are:
laziness and fanaticism.
Don't overdo (that's fanatic).
Don't quit too soon (that's lazy).
Use common sense.

Stretch in the Morning

If you want to have a good day, be sure to s-t-r-r-r-e-t-c-h in the morning!

Here's an excellent set of exercises to do first thing in the morning. It will loosen up your spine, get your kundalini working in your higher energy centers and get you ready to face the day. Do it very consciously, linking your mind and your breath with mantra (**SAT NAM** is highly recommended) for maximum effectiveness.

Of course, you start by chanting
ONG NAMO GURU DEV NAMO.

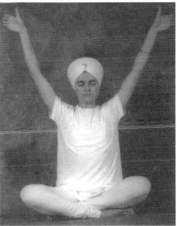

1. **Ego Buster.** Sit in Easy Pose, stretch your arms up and out at a 60 degree angle—really stretch—and don't let your elbows bend. Thumbs stretched up towards the sky with the other fingertips curled onto the mounds at the base of the fingers. Breath of Fire for 2 minutes. Relax 30 seconds to 1 minute.

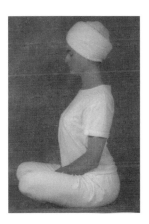

2. **Camel Ride.** Sit in Easy Pose, put your hands on your shins. Flex your spine for 2 minutes. Be sure to move with a continuous fluid motion, without jerking or pausing on the inhalation or the exhalation. Imagine your spine is as limber and loose as a wet noodle, or a rubber band. Straighten out your arms as you inhale and lift your chest, pulling in your lower spine. When you exhale, relax the shoulders forward and extend the spine outward. Relax.

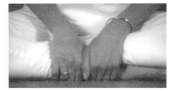

245

STRETCH IN THE MORNING

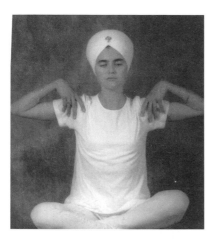

3. Sit in Easy Pose. Hold onto your knees and flex your spine. This time you're working a little higher on the spine. Consciously send the breath into the spine while you keep your eyes focused at the Third Eye point. 2 minutes. Relax.

4. **Spine Flex**. Sit in Easy Pose. Put your hands on your shoulders, fingers in front and thumbs behind. Feel the stretch in your arm pits. Flex your spine for 2 minutes. Inhale, hold the breath briefly while you direct your mind to travel up and down the spine. Exhale and relax.

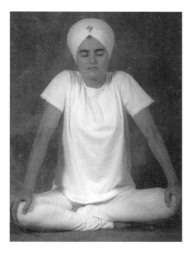

5. **SHOULDER SHRUGS**. Sit in Easy Pose. Inhale, thinking **SAT**, as you lift your shoulders up and exhale thinking **NAAM** as you drop them down. Try to make your shoulders touch your ears, but no cheating, you can't move your head! Continue for 2 minutes. Relax.

6. Sit in Easy Pose. Breathing deeply, drop your chin to your chest, roll it slowly toward one shoulder, then drop your head back and continue circling around. Do this at least five times in one direction, then go in the opposition direction five times, making deep circles with your head around your neck. 2-3 minutes. Inhale deeply, face forward. Exhale and relax.

STRETCH IN THE MORNING

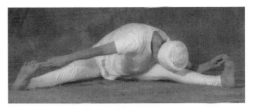

7. Sitting down, legs spread wide apart, grab hold of toes. Inhale sit up in center, exhale bringing your nose down to your left knee (or as far as you can reach, even if it's only a centimeter!) then inhale up to the center and exhale down to the right side. Continue alternating. This is a good spine stretch; it also stretches the nerve that runs up the inside of the thighs. Continue 3 minutes.

8. **"Bird" exercise.** Sit in Easy Pose. Stretch your arms straight out to sides, palms down. Inhale and bring the arms up so the backs of the hands meet over the top of your head then exhale and bring the arms down to the position parallel with the shoulders. Breathe powerfully. Inhale think **SAT**, exhale think **NAAM**. 2 minutes. Relax. This works on the 8th chakra, strengthening your Aura.

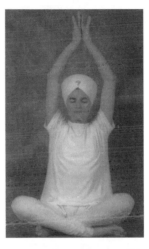

9. **Sat Kriya**. (See Kriya for Elevation, exercise 10.) 2 minutes.

10. Sit in Easy Pose, eyes closed, meditate at the brow point, body relaxed, spine straight. Chant long **SAT NAAM** for 7 minutes, then sit silently and hear the sound of the mantra in your mind.

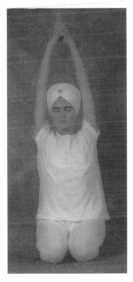

Relax completely for 5 to 10 minutes on your back, in corpse pose, arms at the sides, palms up. (Keep your body in a straight line, do not cross your ankles.) Then stretch left and right, rock on your spine and slowly rise up and greet the day!

Breathe and Move
in the Morning

1. Sitting in Easy Pose, lock your fingers behind your neck. Put any loose hair outside the finger lock so that your fingers touch your neck. Close your eyes. Inhale deeply, hold a few seconds, exhale with force through your nose and hold out a few seconds. Repeat.

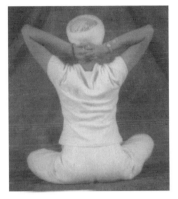

2. Same posture. Immediately begin Breath of Fire. 2 to 5 minutes. Inhale deeply and focus on any part of the body where you want to circulate the healing pranic energy. Exhale and relax briefly. Sit quietly, eyes closed, breathe normally but be intensely aware of the breath flowing in and out of your nostrils. 1 to 2 minutes.

3. Sit in Easy Pose with your spine erect, the rest of the body relaxed. Interlace your fingers behind your back in Venus Lock. Bend forward and touch your forehead to the ground. If you cannot reach from Easy Pose, sit on your heels and bend forward so you can touch your forehead to the ground. Keeping the fingers interlocked, lift the arms straight up as high as possible toward the sky. Hold the position and chant **"ONG"** continuously, inhaling deeply between each repetition. This posture is "Yoga Mudra." Chanting in this position helps to capture the mind. After 1 to 2 minutes, inhale and slowly sit up. Then lie down on your back in corpse pose, arms at the sides, palms up. Relax for 1 minute.

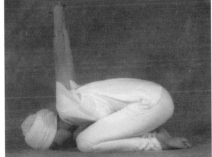

249

BREATHE AND MOVE IN THE MORNING

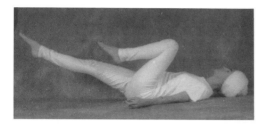

4. Lying on your back, lift both feet up twenty-four inches from the ground and bend alternate knees into the chest, bringing one knee in while the other leg extends out. Continue alternating with a "push-pull" motion, keeping both heels parallel to the ground at the twenty-four inch height. This picks up the pranic energy. 1 to 3 minutes. This exercise MUST be done following exercise # 3.

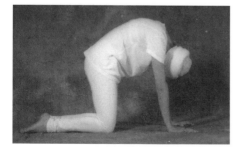

5. **Cow and Cat.** Plant your arms and legs firmly so that you are on all fours, with your hands directly under your shoulders, fingers pointing forward. Your body is positioned like a table, with everything at right angles. Heels together, knees apart about 12 inches. The arms from shoulder to wrist are straight and do not move. The legs from knees to hips are straight and do not move. Inhale as you lift your head up into cow, exhale when head goes down into cat. Inhale SAT, exhale NAM. Start slowly and gradually increase the pace until you can alternate rapidly between lifting the head up while the spine slumps down (cow) and raising the spine up (like an angry cat) while the head goes down. Eyes remain open. 1 to 3 minutes.

Cow and Cat can "make your eyes glitter with a special light." It's also been said (by Yogi Bhajan, of course) that this exercise virtually polishes all your vertabrae!

6. Relax completely in Corpse Pose. 10 to 15 minutes.

Sweat and Laugh
in the Morning (or Anytime!)

ONG NAMO GURU DEV NAMO

1. WARM UP — WAKE UP

a. Navel point: **Stretch Pose—**
Breath of Fire 1 minute.

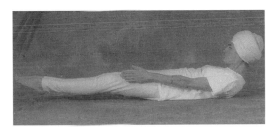

b. **Elimination:** Knees to chest, nose into knees, arms wrapped around legs, hands in Venus Lock. Breath of Fire 1 minute.

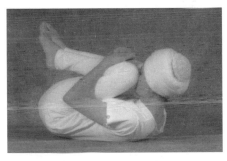

c. **Circumvent Force Builder (Ego Buster):** Sitting in Easy Pose, arms extended out to sides up at 60 degree angle, fingers pressed on mounds of each hand, thumbs up, no bend in elbows, eyes closed, fixed at Third Eye point. Breath of Fire 1 minute. (Practice building up time of these exercises to 3 minutes each.)

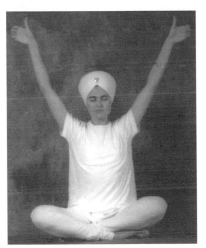

251

SWEAT AND LAUGH IN THE MORNING

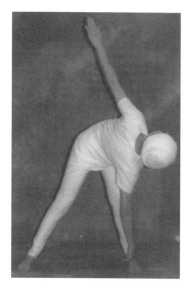

2. STRETCH AND LIMBER UP

a. **Windmill.** Stand with legs approximately 2 feet apart. Stretch your arms straight out to the sides at shoulder level. Inhale in this center position then exhale and bend over touching your right hand to your left foot; inhale up to the center, and exhale down touching your left hand to your right foot. Continue bending to alternate sides for a total of 30 bends (15 on each side). Try to work up to 50. Stand still and relax for 1 minute.

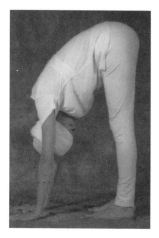

b. **Forward/Back Bends.** Stand erect with your feet about 12 inches apart, exhale as you bend forward touching the palms of your hands to the floor; inhale bringing your arms straight up in front of you and over your head, bending back as far as you can,

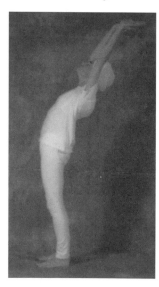

bending the body from the waist. Keep the upper arms close to your ears throughout. 20 times. Relax briefly standing.

SWEAT AND LAUGH IN THE MORNING

c. **Side Bends.** Stand straight with legs 12 inches apart, bring your right arm up in an arc curved over your head toward the left, as you bend your body to the left, keeping your left arm down at your side. Exhale as you bend sideways then inhale up to the center, exhale as you bend to the right, bringing your left arm up over your head in an arc toward the right. It's a graceful movement, like a ballet position. Remember to inhale to the center and exhale as you bend to alternate sides. 30 bends.

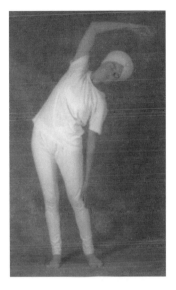

3. Immediately lie down on your back and **LAUGH** as loud as you can for 1 full minute.

4. Relax completely 2 minutes.

5. **Cobra.** Palms of the hands are under your shoulders, fingers facing forward. Lift your chin up first and let your upper body follow. Ideally your heels stay together and your hips and legs remain on the floor while your upper body is arched up with your head back so you could look at the sky - if your eyes were open. Ideally there is no bend in your elbows. This is the ideal. But if you can't do it

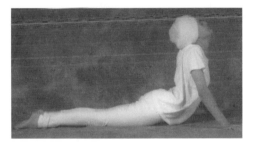

perfectly, don't worry, just do the best you can. Slowly, slowly, flexibility will increase with practice. In this exercise remind yourself to breathe powerfully.

a. Inhale into Cobra. Eyes are closed, focused at Third Eye.

b. Exhale and push your body back bringing the lower torso back into sitting position on the knees with arms outstretched in front of you, keeping your palms flat on floor and stretching your arms as you push back: Total 10 times. Relax briefly on your stomach. Turn your head to one side.

SWEAT AND LAUGH IN THE MORNING

c. Inhale into Cobra, open your eyes wide and try to look at your heels as you inhale turning your head to the left and exhale turning your head to the right. Take full, deep breaths. Total 5 times each side.

d. In Cobra, keeping your eyes wide open, locate a spot on the ceiling as far back as you can see, hold this position keeping your eyes open wide. (Try not to blink—just let them water, it's OK.) Breath-of-Fire for 1 minute.

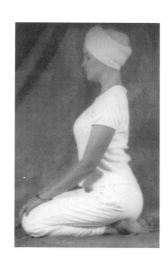

6. **Spine Flexes**
a. Sit on your heels, hands resting on your thighs with the palms down. Inhale, lift your chest high, exhale and collapse the waist, and diaphragm, and shoulders. Flex your spine, total 108 times. (Beginners 1 minute) Inhale think **SAT**. Exhale think **NAAM**.

7. Long deep relaxation in Corpse Pose.

Exercises for Digestion and Elimination

*I*n the chapter about food we explained that even though you may be eating wonderful food, unless you are digesting it properly and eliminating promptly (within 18-24 hours) what the body doesn't use to build blood, and bone, and tissue, you aren't going to be as healthy as you should be. Here is a set of exercises designed especially to help you gain control of your digestive system.

The first kriya is actually called: "How to eliminate from your system at your command."

1. **Vatskar Douti Kriya.** Yogi Bhajan told us that this is a typical "secret" exercise taught by the yogis. It can lead to mastery of the digestive system, and "that will make you very happy!" Here are the conditions:

➤ You have to do it regularly, without missing even one day.

Sit in easy pose, hands on knees. Make a round beak of your mouth and drink in as much air as you can into your stomach in short, continuous "sips"— i.e., short inhalations. When you can't inhale any more, close your mouth and hold your breath in as you roll your stomach left and right as long as possible with neck lock applied. (Chin is pulled straight back.) Churn the stomach area, pulling the navel back and around, left and right. When you can hold the breath in no longer, slowly and gently (not powerfully) exhale through the nose in one continuous stream. Then repeat the exercise two more times (three times total).

➤ Always do this Kriya on an empty stomach.

➤ Do not do it more than twice per day.

255

EXERCISES FOR DIGESTION AND ELIMINATION

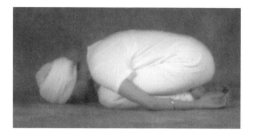

2. Sit on your heels. Bring your forehead to the ground. Keep your hands behind you, resting on the ground. Imagine that you have a big tail and wag it. Move your hips powerfully. Imagine the tail weighs 100 lbs. and you are trying to break the wall behind you. Keep your hips moving for 2 to 3 minutes. Then lie down on your back and rest for 5 minutes. This exercise strengthens the heart.

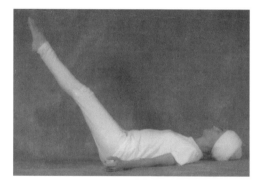

3. Lie down. Press your toes forward. Lift your legs up three feet from the ground. Start Long Deep Breathing. When you can't hold up, come down and then immediately go up and try again. Keep up for 2 minutes. "It will be painful, but this is best for you." This exercise works on the gall bladder and slims the waistline. Relax.

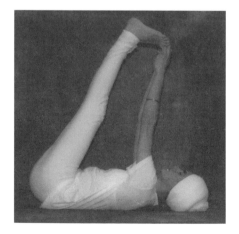

4. Lie down. Bring your legs overhead, catch hold of your toes and roll back and forth from the base of your spine to the back of your neck. Keep holding on to your toes and keep moving. (3 minutes.) You are working on your nervous system and circulation.

EXERCISES FOR DIGESTION AND ELIMINATION

5. Sit up immediately in Sukhasan (Easy cross-legged posture). As calmly as possible, make a "U" of your right hand. Close your right nostril with the thumb of your right hand and use the little finger to close the left nostril. Inhale left, exhale right. Continue. Feel energy going in, disease and sickness going out. 3 minutes.

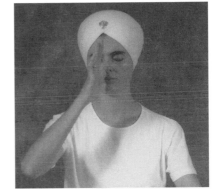

6. Sit in Sukhasan, clasping your hands in bear grip at chest level. Turn your head left and right, keeping the chin parallel to the floor. Inhale as the chin goes over to your left shoulder, exhale as it turns right. This simple exercise works on the thyroid and parathyroid glands, the guardians of health and beauty.

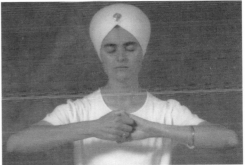

7. Refresh yourself. Sit in easy pose, arms out parallel to the ground. Swing your arms backward in a rolling motion, as if swimming. Make big circles. Then inhale and bend your elbows to bring your hands up to hold your shoulders. This remagnetizes the electric current. While the breath is held, the energy starts circulating. Exhale and let the energy flow to all parts of your body and you will feel refreshed.

Aging doesn't start with years, it starts with deficiency.

8. Lie down flat on your back and relax deeply for 10 minutes or longer.

257

How to Give a Foot Massage

*T*his isn't the only way to give a foot massage, but it's the way Yogi Bhajan first taught us. And, if you're a novice, it will get you started.

Sit on the edge of your bed (or, if you're more comfortable, you can sit in your usual meditation place on the floor, cross-legged) and bring one foot up onto the thigh of the other leg until you can look at the sole of your foot. Then proceed as follows:

You may like to use some massage oil or cream. Try to avoid products with lots of chemicals. Almond oil is excellent. Scented or plain is just fine. Put a towel under your feet so you don't get oil on anything.

Mentally put yourself into a "healing" mode, and realize that the life force that flows through you and through your hands is a Divine gift. It's called "prana." (See the meditation "Healing Hands" to increase pranic energy transfer in your hands.) Put a little bit of oil in the palm of one hand (not too much) and rub it between your hands and then you're ready to apply it to the feet.

Refer to the Foot Chart on page 260 while massaging your feet. Note that the picture on the right side of the page is a diagram of your left foot, and the picture on the left is a diagram of your right foot!

Find the dot on the chart that shows the location of the pituitary gland on the big toe (the nerve ending that corresponds to it, certainly not the gland itself, we know). Apply major pressure with your thumb to that spot on the foot you're going to work on first. You will probably be holding that foot with your other hand, and that is fine. You can massage the pituitary gland location with a strong circular motion with your thumb for a few seconds.

Grasp the base of the big toe with the thumb and forefinger of one hand and using a twisting motion, massage in between the big toe and the next toe. Then pull with an upward motion, as if trying to remove the toe from its socket. It won't come out — I hope. Next, move up about a third of the way (to the

259

FOOT CHART
A guide for basic foot massage

Relaxation of the entire nervous system is possible with proper foot massage. This is because all 72,000 nerves in the body have the endings in the feet. When there is a problem in any area of the body, the corresponding area (as shown in the chart) in the foot will become crystallized with calcium and acid deposits. These crystals must be broken up with foot massage given with 15 to 25 pounds of pressure applied in a circular motion with the fingers and especially the thumbs.

Skin is like a third lung, and you take in pranic energy (life energy) through the pores of the skin as well as through breathing. It is essential to keep the feet clean and best to wear open shoes when possible. Before sleep at night the feet can be washed in cold water and a massage given to calm and relax the nerves. Use a pumice stone to scrub the feet and keep them smooth and free from callouses. Almond oil is especially good for use in massage. Whatever oil or cream you use on your skin, remember it is absorbed by the pores into the bloodstream.

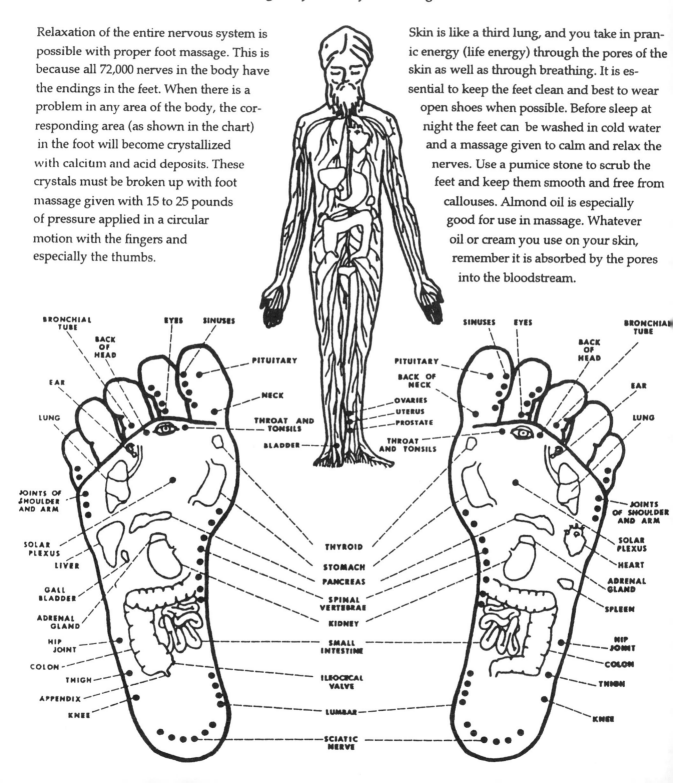

middle of the height of the big toe) and twist again several times, and pull in an upwards motion. Move up again almost to the top of the toe and twist and pull as before. Imagine each toe to be divided into three sections. Proceed on to the next toe and twist and pull as you did on the big toe. Continue until you've worked on all the toes of that foot.

Use your thumbs, fingers, even your knuckles. The object of all this is to stimulate every nerve ending in the soles of your feet (72,000 of them). In order to cover every square centimeter of the surface of your feet, start directly under the big toe, and work your way across the foot in a slow and powerful circular motion until you reach the base of the little toe. Then move down and massage your way back across to the other side. It's like mowing the lawn, or vacuuming a rug. Go left and right, right and left from one side of the foot to the other, moving downward one row at a time to the heel, "leaving no stone unturned." Because you may find "stones" or what seem like rocks as you're massaging! That is, places where there are calcium and acid deposits you can feel. It's a sort of "crunchiness" under your fingers. Return to those spots periodically to work on them some more.

As it says in the foot chart, any place where there is a problem in the body will show up in its corresponding location on the foot. If, for instance, you want to work on your digestive system, spend more time in the area of your intestines and your stomach as shown on the diagram.

Although most of the organs and glands have corresponding nerve endings in both feet, the liver and the heart pressure points are only located in one foot; the heart in the left and the liver in the right. Your appendix seems also to be only accessible from the right foot. Spleen in the left foot, gall bladder in the right. The best thing to do is massage both feet completely, and you won't miss anything. In fact, a word of caution: Always massage both feet. Don't stop after completing one foot, because you will be unbalanced.

A satisfactory foot massage will take at least ten or fifteen minutes. A good one will take about thirty minutes (fifteen minutes each foot); and a super deluxe wonderful foot massage could take as much as one hour.

Do massage the ankles on either side of the Achilles tendon, and then briefly squeeze and release that tendon at least once.

261

Here are a couple of "refinements" to add to your foot massage routine:

➤ Hold all the toes in your hand and flex them forward and back.

➤ Massage up and down an imaginary line running from the middle of the heel to directly underneath the toes (the spot where the bronchial tube is shown). This is a "life-line"; it includes your kidneys.

➤ Knead the feet, as a baker kneads bread dough.

➤ To finish each foot, pat the sole briskly with the palm of your hand (sounds like applause — I love it), then using both hands, starting at the heel, gently draw your fingers up both sides of the foot (top and sole) as if pulling out any remaining tension - ending by pulling up and away from the top of the toes, and then shake your hands out to get rid of it. Be careful not to spill on anyone!

If you are giving someone else a foot massage, it's considerate to keep the foot that you're not working on covered with a towel or blanket, in case it's chilly. If the person falls asleep during the foot massage, don't stop. Keep on until you have completed both feet. It is a sign of success to have someone fall asleep while you are massaging her feet. It indicates that you have really relaxed her completely, and she is probably in the deep sleep stage!

Of course, there are other ways to give a foot massage than the sequence I've listed. But it's a good way to start. It's the way Yogi Bhajan taught us. As you do more foot massage, your intuition will guide you. You will become more aware and sensitive to how much pressure to apply, where and when.

Things to Do at Bedtime

MEDITATION BEFORE BED

This is an excellent self-healing meditation.

The control of the rhythm of the breath in this meditation helps strengthen your nervous system and encourages calm, relaxed sleep. It has been said to help jet-lag and other types of travel fatigue.

Sit in easy pose, spine straight, right hand on top of left hand, palms up. Tips of thumbs are touching. Eyes should concentrate on the tip of the nose. To locate the tip of your nose, hold your forefinger about 6 inches in front of your face, keep looking at it, and bring it to touch the tip of your nose. There, you've got it! Put your finger down, but keep your eyes (which are 9/10 closed) focused on the tip of the nose. (If you're not used to looking at the tip of your nose, it may feel awkward, but in about one minute the nerves will adjust. Keep trying.) Your main mental concentration should be at the brow point (third eye). This stimulates the area between the pineal and the pituitary.

Breathing only through the nose, divide each inhalation into four small, distinct "sniffs." Silently repeat one syllable in your mind with each "sniff" as you inhale in four parts:

SA-TA-NA-MA

Hold the breath in for sixteen counts as you mentally repeat:

SA-TA-NA-MA   SA-TA-NA-MA   SA-TA-NA-MA   SA-TA-NA-MA

Exhale in two parts:

WHA—GURU

Continue for 11 to 15 minutes.

(You can gradually increase time up to 31 minutes.)

263

Then inhale deeply, and exhale completely three times. Immediately inhale deeply and hold the breath as you raise your arms up and out to a 60-degree angle, like the branches of a tree. Hold briefly, exhale and lower them. Repeat this closing sequence twice more, for a total of three times. Relax.

If you do this meditation for thirty-one minutes every night before you go to bed, your sleep will adjust itself to this breath rhythm. After one and a half years, your cycle will become this rhythm.

BEDTIME EXERCISES

To help prepare you for deep sleep, try these three exercises at bedtime. (Of course these may be done at other times in conjunction with exercises for other benefits.)

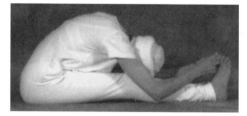

1. **Life-nerve stretch:** Sit with your legs stretched straight out in front, bend forward and grab onto your toes. If you can't reach them, then aim for the ankles, calves, or wherever you can hold on without letting your knees bend. Try to keep the backs of the knees flat on the floor, and your forehead down as close as possible to the knees. Str-r-r-e-e-e-e-t-c-h. Pull back on your toes if you can and keep stretching as you breathe long and deep through your nose, inhaling **SAT** exhaling **NAM**.

The life-nerve (which runs up the back of your legs) affects your emotional balance and nervous system, and this exercise even works on your digestive system. No set time, but about three minutes is recommended. You can end by inhaling deeply, exhaling completely and applying the Mul Bandh.

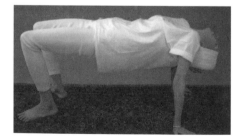

2. **Bridge Pose** is included in a much longer set of exercises, printed in the *Sadhana Guidelines* manual that was taught by Yogi Bhajan specifically to work on sleep problems. That excellent set is called "How to Conquer Sleep". Plant your palms and feet firmly on the ground and keep your arms and legs at right

angles to the floor. No bend in the elbows. Support your body so that from your knees to your shoulders you are in a straight line parallel to the floor. You can let your head fall back. Your hands are shoulder width apart, knees and feet are also apart about that same distance. Everything is at right angles so that your body forms a "bridge" — that must be where they got the name. Again, you're working on the nervous system. Apply Root Lock (Mul Bandh) and hold, with normal breathing, 1 to 3 minutes, then breathe long and deep for another minute or two or three.

3. Lie flat on your back. Breathe long and deep for about 30 seconds, then on the next inhalation, stretch your hands up to the sky as if reaching for the moon, stretch from the shoulders and really reach, grab onto the prana of the universe, and slowly, with the breath still held in, bend your fingers into your palms to form fists. Then still holding the breath, bend your elbows and slowly bring the fists down toward the center of your chest, and exhale when you reach it. Pull as if you are resisting an opposing force. Your arms will shake. Repeat the exercise one more time.

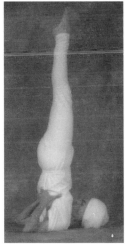

4. **Shoulder Stand** is done by lying flat on the back, placing the hands under the hips for support as you first lift both legs up to 90 degrees and then use your hands under your hips to push your body up till the toes are pointing to the ceiling and the body is in as straight a line as you can manage. Your weight is balanced on the triangle of your elbows, upper arms, and shoulders. Your head remains on the floor. Hold the position for 1 to 3 minutes, with long deep breathing. Slowly unwind, and come down to lie flat on your back. Relax.

GOOD NIGHT!

GOD BLESS YOU

Three Meditations to Eliminate Stress

Here are three important meditations to share with your family and friends, your enemies, your neighbors, your grocer or your dry-cleaner!

Here are three dynamite kriyas that are designed to work on the number one killer in our nation: STRESS. If you want to feel relaxed and mellow, practice these three unusual meditations.

Yogi Bhajan gave them on November 18, 1991, at the Whole Life Expo in Los Angeles. He told everyone in the audience to teach them freely to everyone, share them with their families and friends, children, everyone. In his class the next night at Yoga West, he told us to do them, and to write them up and send them to everyone — no restrictions. So here they are, no holds barred! Share them with your friends and your enemies, teach them to your neighbors and your in-laws, your grocer and your dry-cleaner!

1 Pittar Kriya. Put your left palm at center of your chest (on heart center); right elbow bent, your right hand, cupped, moves past your right ear, as if throwing water back behind you over your shoulder. Keep the right arm moving back and forth, making sure that the wrist passes the right ear, for 11 minutes. Set a timer, or watch a clock, because the time is to be exact. Not less, not more. Then inhale deeply, hold the breath while pressing the arm as far back behind you as possible. (Repeat the inhale and hold twice more.) This Kriya is to eliminate stress and clean the liver.

2   This is for the glandular system and brings all the Chakras into balance: Bend your elbows and press them in at the rib cage, and with your palms facing up, hold onto the first joint of the Saturn (middle) fingers of each hand with the thumbs, and then release quickly with a jerk, meanwhile chanting rapidly aloud in a monotone, "**HAR , HAR.** " with each flick of the fingers, over and over again using the tip of the tongue. Continue this rapid 'flicking' motion. (The "a" in "har" is a short sound, pronounced like the first syllable in "a-gain" and the "r" is rolled.) Eyes are fixed at the tip of the nose.

After 11 minutes, inhale deeply and hold the breath, while continuing to capture and then release the tip of the Saturn finger with the same springing motion. Exhale and inhale again, hold the breath and keep the fingers moving. (Repeat the breath inhalation and retention once more, for a total of three times.) The thumb represents the "Id."

3   For your Nervous System (sympathetic, parasympathetic and central nervous systems): Works on your ability to DO — gets rid of your "junk." Gets rid of "madness." Look at the tip of your nose. Extend your arms out straight to both sides, keep them straight (no bend in elbows), palms down — and criss-cross them in front of you, horizontally, over and under while chanting **HAR** continuously, consciously using the tip of the tongue each time the arms cross.

After 11 minutes, inhale deeply, hold the breath while you continue to move the arms. (Repeat the breath inhalation and retention twice more, relax.)

COLD SHOWERS

Yogi Bhajan reminded everyone about COLD SHOWERS for hydro-therapy. They open the capillaries. You have to go in and out of the water about four times — until the water no longer feels cold, meanwhile massaging your body. Someone asked about taking a hot shower first, and then ending with cold water. He replied, "That is like eating a lot of junk food and then having a healthy meal."

268

Take Care of Yourself
As a Woman

Your achievement in life is based on your glandular secretion. The body could last for 120 years were it not for glandular imbalance. To keep the glands in shape:

➤ Eat nurturing food

➤ Take cold showers to flush the capillaries

➤ Sweat 15 minutes a day so that glands can secrete

➤ Your food should be properly seasoned and seasonal

➤ Wait four hours after eating before going to bed...

KUNDALINI YOGA FOR WOMEN

"No woman's body has to become ugly. Woman can get out of shape and then get back in shape. The body has an automatic inner capacity towards that. So don't blame the body. The fact is, woman must exercise." — Yogi Bhajan

There are certain exercises in Kundalini Yoga that are particularly valuable for women to practice.

"THE MAGNIFICENT SEVEN"

These seven exercises were recommended by Yogi Bhajan at KWTC in 1988 as a daily practice for every woman to "maintain her youth and beauty."

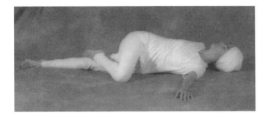

1a. **Cat Stretch.** Stretch to both sides. See Illustration.

1b. **Eye Opener.** "Wake up your eyes in your hands" as described in *How to Get Up in the Morning.*

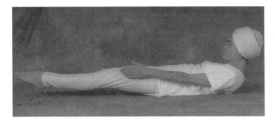

2. **Stretch Pose** with Breath of Fire for 10 to 15 seconds. *(See page 117 for instructions.)*

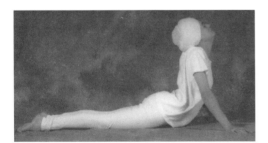

3. **Cobra Pose.** Hands under shoulders. Fingers pointing forward. Use your arms to press your upper body up and lock your elbows straight. Pick a point on the ceiling and fix your gaze on it. Long Deep Breathing or Breath of Fire 1 minute.

4. **Cat and Cow.** A natural fluid movement of the spine, neck and head. Inhale as the spine goes up (like an angry cat) and exhale as you slump it down. The head goes opposite to the spine. Breathe powerfully. Speed can be increased as flexibility is gained.

5. **Mental Standard.** "...and there is another hygiene. It is called mental standard. Three times during the day to check your mental strength, sit down and stretch your legs straight. Hold your toes in your hands. Touch your nose to your knees. Anytime you feel tense, that much you are off the energy, you need to balance it. If you want to face the world twelve hours, do this exercise every four hours. For a female, this is a must!"

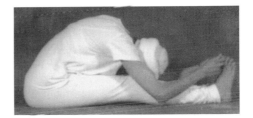

6a. **Rock Pose.** Sit on your heels. Breath of Fire or Long Deep Breathing for 5 minutes.

6b. **Rock Pose on Your Back.** "Whenever you eat, you must sit on your heels for 5 to 7 minutes. And if it is possible for you in your life, in the evening sometime, lie down like this flat on your back. If a woman can do this posture in the evening time, she will hardly get sick. The time is between 5 to 7 minutes. And, for the best results, it is to be done in the evening time - in the twilight zone, when the sun is setting, it's the best."

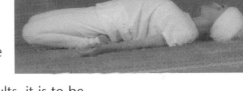

7. **Shoulder Stand.** One posture, Gurpreet Karni Kriya (Shoulder Stand) is especially good for the female. From a prone position on your back, raise your legs up to 90 degrees and then raise the entire torso up to 90 degrees, making the body form a straight line from shoulders to toes. Support the weight of your body on your elbows and shoulders using your hands to support the lower spine. The chin is pressed into the chest. Hold for 5 minutes in the morning. Shoulder Stand releases pressure on all the organs and stimulates the thyroid gland. Every woman should do this posture for 5 to 7 minutes... "Health-wise, hygienic-wise you will be in good shape."

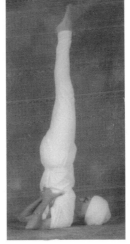

A CONSCIOUS ACT !

It is important and very beneficial for every woman to exercise each day. It is this conscious act of working on ourselves that gives us a beauty, radiance, and grace. The following exercises should be done regularly to keep the spine, organs, and nervous system strong and healthy. You have already learned most of them in previous sets.

1. **Rock Pose.** Sitting on heels, palms on thighs or hands relaxed on lap, spine straight, relaxed. Excellent for digestion. I read a quaint note somewhere that said if a woman brushes her hair every day, sitting in rock pose, Vajrasan, she will never get gray hair! I don't vouch for it, but it seemed an interesting possibility.

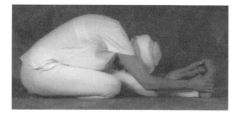

2. **Life Nerve Stretch.** Sit on your right heel, left leg extended straight out, and draw your forehead to the left knee. Hold onto your toes (making sure to keep the backs of the knees on the floor) with Long Deep Breathing for 1 to 2 minutes then change sides. (Or, instead of sitting on each foot, draw it into the groin and then pull your forehead down to your knee.) Finish by extending both legs in front holding onto your ankles or your toes.

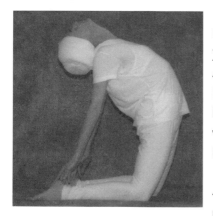

3. **Camel Pose.** (This is not "camel ride.") Come up onto your knees with your thighs perpendicular to the floor. Arch back, holding onto your heels. Let your head fall back, press your hips forward and hold the position with Long Deep Breathing. Camel Pose adjusts the reproductive organs.

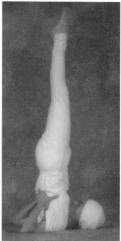

4. **Shoulder Stand.** Explained on page 265.

272

5. **Archer Pose.** Stand firmly with the right leg extended forward, the knee bent, carrying the weight of the body. Left leg is straight out behind you, foot planted firmly. (It will be easier to balance if you turn the back foot out somewhat, at about a 45 degree angle.) Your right arm is extended straight out in front of you, as if you are holding a bow, and your left arm is pulled back, as if pulling an arrow taut on the bowstring. Feel this stretch across the chest. Keep your eyes open, staring straight ahead. Steady, hold the position with Long, Deep Breathing, 5 minutes on each side. The deeper the knee bend, the better.

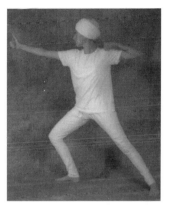

6. **Baby Pose.** Sit on your heels. Bring your forehead to the floor in front of you. Arms remain relaxed at your sides with palms facing up, near your feet. Relaxed breath, 2 to 5 minutes. Baby Pose brings needed circulation to the eyes, ears, nose, and throat.

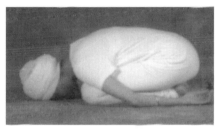

7. **Bow Pose.** Lying on your stomach, take hold of your ankles and pull up, raising the thighs and head as high as possible, creating an arch in your spine. Hold the position with Long, Deep Breathing for 2 to 3 minutes. (Bow Pose is sometimes done with Breath of Fire.)

Bow Posture is very beneficial to a woman's mind. It has the ability to bring peace to the mind. A woman must also learn Sat Kriya, how to chant with breathing rhythm in certain postures, and the **Sa-Ta-Na-Ma** meditation. These are essential for a woman's glandular system. **Sa-Ta-Na-Ma** meditation is especially recommended for every woman.

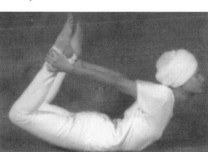

273

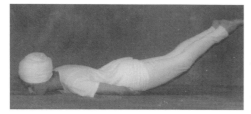

8. **Locust Pose.** Lie on your stomach. Make your hands into fists and place them under your hips, just above the leg-joints. Hold your heels together. Keeping your chin on the floor, raise your legs up off the floor and hold the position with Long Deep Breathing for 1 to 2 minutes

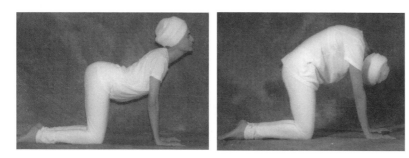

9. **Cow Pose.** Hold the position with Long Deep Breathing 2 to 3 minutes.

10. **Cat Pose.** Hold the position with Long Deep Breathing 2 to 3 minutes.

11. **Stretch Pose** is so basic and necessary, it shows up everywhere! It adjusts the navel point, strengthens the reproductive organs and glands, and energizes the whole body. *(See page 117 for instructions.)*

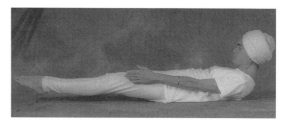

12. **Corpse Pose.** Yes, this is an "exercise," every bit as important as any of the others, and in some ways, more important! Relaxation is not a luxury, it is a necessity in our lives, and lying in corpse pose helps the body relax completely. Be sure that the body is in a straight line and that your palms are turned upward as you're lying on your back. To relax the mind as well, focus on your breathing, thinking **SAT** as you inhale, and **NAAM** as you exhale.

13. **Sat Kriya.** Here's the "grand finale." *(See page 233.)* Sat Kriya is unusual in our practice of Kundalini Yoga, because although it does begin to work within less than a minute, the time can be increased up to 31 minutes if you're game and really want maximum strength! SAT KRIYA works on just about everything in the body, as well as the mind and the emotions. It drives away depression, raising your kundalini to the higher chakras.

274

DISEASE PREVENTION FOR WOMEN

Here's a simple set of six you can do to vary your routine. Relax briefly after each exercise and at the end of the set.

1. Lie on your back. Connect the little finger and thumb of each hand and criss-cross your arms (keep the arms straight) back and forth over your chest. 2 minutes.

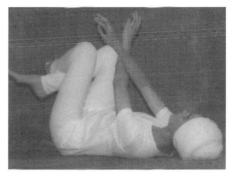

2. Keep your arms moving as in #1, pull your knees up and criss-cross your lower legs from side to side (left to right and right to left). 2 minutes.

3. Still lying on your back, with your arms and legs relaxed and your head on the floor, turn your head from side to side rapidly. 2 minutes.

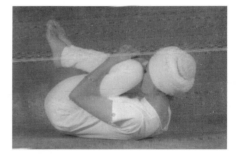

4. Bring your knees to your chest, wrap your arms around them and lift your head up so your nose is in between your knees. Hold the position and do Breath of Fire powerfully for 1 minute.

5. Turn over onto your stomach and beat your rear end with your fists. This is to keep you youthful, it's not a punishment! 2 minutes.

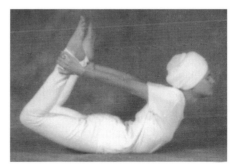

6. Come into Bow Pose and balance on your navel. Hold the position and do Breath of Fire. 2 minutes.

THE POWER OF FOODS

For Women Only
(in Yogi Bhajan's words)

"Food must be approved by your nose and taste good or it will take seven days and maximum energy to get it out of the body, cutting the blood supply to the brain and extremities, even affecting memory."

These foods are good for men, too, but they are especially beneficial for women.

DEPRESSION PREVENTION

"If you take one banana early in the morning, and at four p.m., one tablespoon of raisins, you should never be depressed. Eat one banana a day for potassium. If you can maintain the level of your potassium you can never falter."

ENERGY

"...If you take a cup of Yogi Tea three times in the day, you won't fall flat. The formula of Yogi Tea *(See Recipe Section)* is for the liver." (It also tastes delicious.) In the early days of 3HO you could always tell a 3HO house by the fragrant aroma of the pot of Yogi Tea boiling merrily away on the stove. (And sometimes boiling over! You have to watch it closely.)

STRENGTH

"One cantaloupe can make a woman fit for a week."

TOXIC CLEAN-UP

"Three days of simply living on watermelon can clean your body as a woman. A man requires eleven days. Look at the tragedy! If a man wants to cleanse himself from all the toxins, he needs to go on a watermelon fast for eleven days minimum. A woman can do it in three days, and she is fine."

MORE GOOD FOODS

- "As many pears as you eat, that much younger you will look. Pears replace the iron deficiency in the blood. *(Ed. Note: Pear juice in particular has been known to help in getting rid of fibroids. Also try cutting pears into small chunks and boiling them in a small amount of water with cinnamon and vanilla. Yummmmm.)*
- Broccoli has the most digestible protein.
- Eat eggplant at least one day per week. It is sexy, full of iron, and when cooked properly, one of the most cleansing foods you can get."

FLYING HIGH

"Take a couple of mangoes early in the morning, add some yogurt, some water, rosewater if possible, blend it into a lassi and drink it—the whole day you will feel like you have wings in your armpits and fly!" *(Ed. Note: Lassi is an Indian drink made of liquified yogurt and flavoring, it is not the famous movie dog. It is pronounced "lussie.")*

YOGIC TIDBITS FOR WOMEN
More Quotes from Yogi Bhajan

CONQUER FATIGUE

Yogi Bhajan says, "When I can't wake up, I don't want to get up, when I am tired beyond my repair capacity and everything has gone wrong, God bless the cold shower! *(Explained in detail in the chapter: How to Get Up in the Morning.)* If you can't take a full cold shower, at least wash your hands, wash your elbows with cold water, wash your face, make your hands wet with cold water and massage your ears. Take a wet hand and put it on your chest and on the lower back. Wash your feet. You'll be fit for another three or four hours. When the body wants to sink in, the cold shower feeds the capillaries with extra blood and gives you a newness." Massage your breasts under the cold water every day to stimulate the circulation. (With the incidence of breast cancer in women over 40 alarmingly high, we need to do everything possible to avoid it. Psychologically it has been linked to inner anger. Which is another major reason to clear out the subconscious with a regular spiritual practice of meditation and mantra. *Sadhana, sadhana, sadhana!*)

MAKE-UP

"You have to learn to shine your face, not to paint it up. You are not warring Indians. Make-up is not to make up for your handicaps. Make-up rather is very open evidence that you are handicapped. Make-up is a declaration." (Yogi Bhajan strongly supports natural beauty. It's true, when your diet is right, and your exercise is right, and your thinking is positive, your face is going to glow naturally. Above all, smile!)

STIMULANTS

"Stimulants kill you. It doesn't matter what they are."

RISE AND SHINE

"You must not jump up (out of bed) like a hot potato out of the pan onto the ground - that is not for you. Men can afford to suffer, you can't. Any woman who jumps up kills her youth that day and suffers that month. That is how your electromagnetic field gets totally messed up.

278

"Just open your eyes in your hand. That will keep your eyes young for a long time. If you open them straight, you will very soon have to wear glasses. Okay now, Cat-stretch left; Cat-stretch right. Next do stretch pose: legs up a little, feet up and hands up and do that for just a few seconds. And now get up slowly. How many of you get up this way? If you do not, ladies, you can get a common cold and grow old very fast."

BUT NOT IN PUBLIC, PLEASE!

"Whenever you eat you must sit on your heels for five to seven minutes afterwards. If it is possible for you, in the evening lie down flat on your back while sitting on your heels. If a woman can do this posture in the evening, she will hardly ever get sick. Between five and seven minutes is a must. For best results, do it in the evening during the twilight zone when the sun is setting. (This is shown in the "Magnificent Seven.")

WASHING YOUR HAIR

"How do you wash your hair? Does anybody know? Water, soap, or shampoo and conditioner? You are wrong. Put oil on your head and massage it to death. Then wrap it with a thick cloth so you may not mess up your clothes. Take oil and yogurt mixed together with the fragrance you want and massage your hair. Make what they call a "towel cloth," which you can tie very tightly so it may not fall off. Let it stay there for an hour or two. After that take your shampoo and wash your hair. Then if you want to blow dry it or not that is your option. The best method is to stay in the sun and let the natural air and sunshine take care of it. Once a week you must expose your hair, head, and skull to the sun. That is a must."

LITTLE BANG THEORY

A woman should never wear her hair over her forehead. God can grow hair wherever He likes, but no hair grows on the forehead. The forehead bone, the sinus bones or the frontal bone, is porous so it can function to transmit light to the pineal gland in the brain. When Ghengis Khan conquered China, he issued orders that all the women must cut their hair and wear bangs over their forehead. He knew this would keep them timid and subjugated. Believe it or not. The point is, you have a choice!

279

GRACE OF GOD Meditation

The technique of positive affirmation has been around for thousands of years. It's nothing new. Words increase in power through repetition, and when you are repeating truth, WOW! the impact is enormous. Yogi Bhajan has given us one of the most powerful affirmations a woman can do. It's called the "Grace of God Meditation," or "GGM" for short.

The GGM meditation is designed to evoke and manifest the inner grace, strength, and radiance of each woman.

The fact is, woman is the Grace of God. Woman is Shakti. The problem is, she doesn't know it. The GGM meditation is designed to evoke and manifest the inner grace, strength, and radiance of each woman. It helps her to tune in directly with the Adi Shakti, the Primal Power within her own being. It empowers a woman to channel her emotions in a positive direction, strengthen her weaknesses, develop mental clarity and effective communication, and gives her the patience to go through the tests of her own karma. It enables her to merge the limited ego into Divine will, as well as to improve her physical health.

By practicing this meditation, a woman's thoughts and behavior, personality and projection become aligned with the infinite beauty and nobility unveiled by the mantra. The amazing thing is, this is such an easy meditation to do! That is why I'm "selling" it so strongly, because you might pass it over because it's so simple, and not realize what a profound effect it can have on your life.

It is definitely a very powerful technique, but all the benefits claimed don't mean a thing unless you do it! So, please practice it faithfully for at least forty days. Sunrise is the best time to do it, and then again at sunset. What a beautiful way to begin and end your day! Five times a day is recommended for women going through menopause. Be sure to do the meditation on an empty stomach.

Part One

Lie down on your back, fully relaxing your face and body. Inhale deeply, hold the breath in while you silently repeat "I am Grace of God" ten times. You can tense your fingers one at a time to keep count. Exhale all the air out, hold it out and repeat the mantra ten

Erase your insecurity!

times with the breath held out. Inhale and continue this process of repeating the mantra ten times on each inhale and ten times on each exhale for a total of five inhalations and five exhalations. This totals one hundred silent repetitions. Then:

Part Two

Relax your breath, and with eyes still closed, slowly come sitting up into easy pose. Bring your right hand into Gyan Mudra (index finger curled under the thumb, other three fingers stretched out straight, palm up, wrist resting on the knee, elbow straight). The left hand is held up by the left shoulder, palm flat and facing forward. This is called the "vow" position. Your hand is held up as if you are taking an oath. Keep the breath relaxed and normal. Tense only one finger of the left hand at a time, keeping the other fingers straight but relaxed. Meditate on the governing energy of that finger *(please refer to illustration)*, then repeat aloud five times, "I am Grace of God." Continue this sequence for each of the remaining fingers, finishing with the thumb.

When both parts of the meditation are completed, lower the left hand down and relax for a few minutes.

Your emotions will become more positively channeled and any physical or mental ill health will be greatly improved. It is said that when you continue practicing for one year your aura will become tipped with

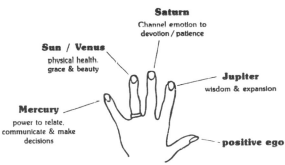

gold or silver, and great strength and God's healing powers will flow through you. "Grace of God meditation will give you self-effectiveness."

Practice the Grace of God meditation twice a day, focusing your concentration on the particular attribute you want to correct or enhance in your life. God bless you!

Recipes

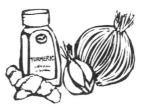

Yogi Tea

Yogi Bhajan's Original Recipe

Copyright Yogi Bhajan 1969 Printed with Permission

You can buy Yogi Tea pre-packaged, loose or in tea-bags, and even in various flavors, but for the most quintessential, excellent, best experience of yogi tea, count out your own spices and make it from scratch! Following is the original recipe as Yogi Bhajan taught it to me in 1969.

Measurements can vary according to your taste. Be careful not to put in too many cloves or cinnamon sticks.

To 3 qts. of boiling water add:
    20 whole cloves, see them dance!
    20 whole green cardamom pods (you can open them up)
    20 whole black peppercorns
    5 sticks of cinnamon

Continue boiling for 15-20 minutes, then add:
    1/4 teaspoon of any black tea. After one or two minutes add:
    1/2 cup cold milk per cup of remaining liquid

When it returns to the boiling point, remove immediately from heat. (Watch closely so it doesn't boil over.) Strain and serve with honey to taste, if desired.

The black pepper is a blood purifier, the cardamom is for the colon, the cloves for the nervous system, and the cinnamon for the bones. The milk aids in the easy assimilation of the spices and avoids irritation to the colon. The black tea acts as an alloy for all of the ingredients, achieving a new chemical structure which makes the tea a healthy as well as delicious drink.

Slices of fresh ginger root may also be included, especially when you are suffering from a cold, recovering from the flu, or you just want extra energy.

Golden Milk

"Snap, crackle, and pop" is not what you want to hear when you bend your knees. Turmeric, that little orange spice, helps make the bones and joints flexible. And it doesn't take much. Here's a recipe to serve that very purpose:

> 1/8 teaspoon turmeric
> 3 cardamom pods (optional)
> 1/4 cup water (approx.)

Simmer 5 to 7 minutes, then add:

> 1 cup milk
> 2 tablespoons almond oil (cold pressed)

Bring just up to the boiling point, do not boil !

If desired, add sweetener (honey or maple syrup) to taste. You can also make it frothy by putting it in the blender - use the lowest setting.

Drink warm. It's a great bedtime drink.

Ginger Tea

Good for everyone! Men, women, and children. Particularly useful for women to drink for energy during menstrual period.

Slice up about one finger-length of ginger root (available in the produce section of grocery stores) and boil in about 1 quart of water for approximately 10 minutes. You don't even have to peel the ginger. Strain, sweeten to taste (or not) add milk (or not), and drink hot. Use honey or maple syrup. Anything but white sugar! That would defeat the whole purpose ot the ginger tea. Ginger root supplies added energy to the nerve centers in the spine.

Kitcheree

High Protein/Easy to Digest
(Based on Yogi Bhajan's recipe)

(Measurements are approximate)

> 16 cups of water
>
> 1/2 cup mung beans

Boil the mung beans first, for about ten minutes, then add the other ingredients

> 1 cup thoroughly washed white basmati rice
>
> 1 onion, chopped
>
> 5 to 7 cloves of garlic, sliced or chopped
>
> 1 teaspoon peeled and chopped ginger root
>
> 1/2 teaspoon turmeric
>
> 1/2 teaspoon ground black pepper
>
> 3/4 teaspoon crushed red chili flakes
>
> 1/2 teaspoon cumin or garam masala (Indian spice—optional)

Boil gently (covered) 30 to 40 minutes until very soft and "soupy."
Add 1 or 2 cups of any chopped vegetables preferably green, such as asparagus, celery, broccoli, zucchini, swiss chard. You can also add carrots and/or mushrooms or you may prefer to keep it very simple and only use one or two green vegetables.

Optional: During the cooking, add Braggs Liquid Aminos (similar to Tamari), about 20 'squirts' for the above recipe should do it, or serve on the side. A few sprigs of fresh mint cooked in with all the vegetables is really good!

Suggestion: For a complete meal, serve with yogurt and toasted Pita Bread!

Find more Yogic Recipes and Vegetarian delights in the *Golden Temple Cookbook* (by Yogi Bhajan), *From Vegetables With Love* (by Siri Ved Kaur), and *A Taste of India* (by Inderjit Kaur).

Potent Potatoes

Here's Yogi Bhajan's original recipe for a delicious dish, almost a meal in itself, incorporating that dynamic herb root trinity: garlic, onions, and ginger. I found it in my notes from 1971.

Bake a potato after washing it in warm water. Meanwhile, saute in olive oil:

  3 ounces finely chopped ginger root
  4 ounces chopped onion
  1 teaspoon (approx.) finely chopped garlic
  A little turmeric
  Caraway seed
  Red pepper (to your taste, watch out, it's HOT)
  Dash of powdered cardamom
  A few cloves
  A sprinkle of powdered cinnamon

Saute until onion is nicely browned. Mix with cottage cheese to your taste. Cut baked potatoes in half lengthwise, scoop out the insides and mash. For each potato half, mix in half of the above mixture with the mashed potato and replace in the potato skins. Put a slice of cheddar cheese on top and melt in the oven. Garnish with fresh pineapple, radishes, and sliced green pepper. These are truly POTENT potatoes! So don't eat more than two at a time. If you do overeat, take a glass of milk and it will cool you down.

Serving suggestion: Serve with salad and a bowl of yogurt. If you're sensitive to dairy, use goat or soy cheese and goat yogurt.

Remember to chant whenever you cook anything. Blessing food was one of the first lessons Yogi Bhajan taught me. Never eat anything without thanking God for providing it, and always chant when you cook. Vibrations do go into the food you are handling. You certainly want to add the blessings of your prayers to anything you are going to serve your family and friends. They will feel it. If you're ever privileged to eat anything cooked by Yogi Bhajan, you'll know what I mean.

288

SPICY BEET-SWEET POTATO CASSEROLE
Yogi Bhajan's own recipe

When the flu season comes around, it's time to eat some special foods. An ounce of prevention is worth a pound of cure! This Beet Casserole tastes wonderful and your liver and your intestines will love you. If you are hypoglycemic, proceed with caution, as beets are very sweet.

Ingredients:

4 medium size beets
1 large sweet potato
1/2 cup water chestnuts
1 large onion, chopped fine
1/4 cup chopped or grated ginger root
5 cloves of garlic, chopped fine
1 jalapeno, chopped (optional)

1 teaspoon turmeric
1 teaspoon cinnamon
1 teaspoon ground black pepper
1 teaspoon cayenne
1/2 teaspoon cardamom powder
1/4 teaspoon clove powder
1/4 teaspoon nutmeg
3 tablespoons ghee (clarified butter)
Braggs Aminos to taste

Steam or pressure cook sweet potato and beets together. Remove potato after 10 minutes of steamed pressure and continue to steam beets for another 10-15 minutes, or until soft.

In a large sauce pan, melt ghee and add chopped onions. After 3-5 minutes, add ginger, garlic, and jalapeno. Continue to saute until onions are well cooked. Cook over medium-low heat so onions will not burn. Once this mixture is well done, add spices and saute over low heat for a few minutes.

Remove beets from steamer, rinse under cold water and remove skin. Remove skin from potato also. Chop potato into small cubes along with beets (the smaller the better). Add this mixture to onions, ginger, and garlic and slowly mix. Add water chestnuts and continue to mix thoroughly. Also if you like, add Braggs to suit your taste.

You may sprinkle freshly chopped cilantro over this beet dish. Best served with Saffron Rice and a hot cup of Yogi Tea! (I like to eat it with yogurt.)

Saffron Rice

Saute about 1/4 teaspoon saffron in a teaspoon of ghee for a few minutes. Add 2 cups of rice to 4 cups of boiling water and cook. You may add some lemon juice to give extra flavor.

Ghee

Ghee is clarified butter. You can make ghee by gently boiling unsalted butter long enough to have the impurities rise to the top of the pan. Keep skimming off this "froth" until you're left with the clear golden liquid ghee. It will harden if refrigerated and keep for a long time, even if not refrigerated.

Sources and Resources

BOOKS

Bookstore shelves are bursting with all kinds of self-help books. There are books on time-management, psychology, philosophy, relationships, metaphysics, astrology, numerology, spirituality, just about every conceivable topic dealing with how to make the most out of life, and how to straighten out the messes people seem to get themselves into.

Some books are really good —- and some are not. In fact some books can be very misleading. Not everything is gospel. Just because something is in print doesn't necessarily guarantee its validity. You have to pan for the gold that is buried in the pages of some of the volumes that come your way. When I was in my early twenties, I began to study Eastern philosophy, attended lectures at the Vedanta Temple in Hollywood as well as at the Self Realization Fellowship (founded by Paramahansa Yogananda) in Hollywood and in the Pacific Palisades. People gave me books on metaphysics and oriental philosophy. I devoured everything I could find that might give me some clue as to the meaning of life. Some books (sometimes only excerpts from them) became lifetime inspiration and guides for me.

If an idea had merit, if it rang true, it seemed to jump right off the page at me. It was as if it were printed in bright, bold, technicolor letters. Something inside me shouted "Yes!" when I read a phrase that rang a bell. This is still the case. Of course, I try to keep in mind that there is always margin for error in the way I interpret an author's words. We usually hear what we want to hear, and see what we want to see. Truth, with a capital "T," isn't always easy to understand, nor to accept.

I love to discover a new way of explaining things that makes concepts clearer. I try never to "throw the baby out with the bath water," but to extract what seems useful and relevant to me, and simply leave the rest behind.

I'd like to suggest to you some of the books that have made the most impact on me. Some of them are new and some of them are timeless classics that I don't believe will ever be outdated. I've read and reread some of them many times. With each reading I learn something new that deepens my understanding.

It is a great pleasure to share the discovery of a great book with a friend. (I hope you will want to tell someone about this book!)

There's a saying, "When the student is ready, the Teacher will appear." Similarly, I think when the student is ready, the right book will appear. I've found that the more I know, the easier it becomes to learn more. I hope these books will serve you as they have served me, adding to your frame of reference and increasing your appreciation of this great adventure called life.

Here goes:

OLDIES BUT GOODIES

PHILOSOPHY

There is a River *by Thomas Sugrue*

(Biography of Edgar Cayce). Not only does this tell the story of Cayce's remarkable, life-transforming experience while under hypnosis, when he tapped into a higher source of knowledge and information for healing,[1] but the part of this book I like to share with people is his detailed description of how God created this creation, out of Himself. Cayce uses the analogy describing God as a vast, shoreless ocean.

An ocean has huge waves in some places, icebergs in others, but whatever its condition, warm or cold, tranquil and serene, or with storms raging and crashing, water is always H_2O. Cayce's analogy affirms the essential unity and oneness of God and all of God's manifestations.

Cosmic Consciousness *by Dr. Richard Bucke*

I call your attention to the first 80 pages or so as "required reading." That is where Dr. Bucke, a Canadian psychiatrist, explains the theory of the evolution of consciousness. The rest of the book is case histories. I found the idea fascinating, that a rock has a basic "consciousness" which enables it to keep its molecular structure intact holding it together as a solid mass. And that consciousness then evolved into the more advanced awareness of plant life, which has the consciousness to seek light and moisture. Plants have the consciousness to turn green, through photo-synthesis. The next step on the consciousness ladder is that of animals, which are at the instinctual level. Higher on the scale, in human beings, intuitive awareness emerges. But that's not the final product of the evolution of consciousness. There is something that goes beyond intuition, and that is what the Masters and Saints and Yogis experience, the transformational state of "Cosmic Consciousness," which we call the state of "Yoga." Although there is no change of form, the beings who evolve in consciousness beyond human consciousness may be as different from you and me as a plant is from a rock, or a man is from a dog!

How To Know God *by Christopher Isherwood and Swami Prabhavananda*

If I were cast away on a desert island, this is one of the books I would definitely want to have with me. I think the perspective it provides is invaluable. It gives a foundation for understanding those impersonal cosmic laws, the "rules of the game" which apply to every event in our personal lives. This understanding can make every moment spiritually meaningful. It takes the sting out of many painful experiences, when they can be looked at as lessons and opportunities for growth - which, of course, they are.

Based on the ancient aphorisms of Patanjali, who was the first Yogi ever to write down the technology of Raj Yoga ("King" or "Royal" Path of Yoga), I consider *How To Know God* a "must have" classic. Its ancient wisdom describes the evolution of a human being, points out his or her potential and how the cycle of birth, death, and reincarnation works. It explains that we are born with certain thought patterns *(samskaras)* already established in our minds and tells how they affect us. It describes the eight steps to Samadhi (enlightenment).

The book is not easy to digest all at once, so the approach I suggest is to read a little at a time. Don't struggle with any concepts that are difficult. Just keep on reading and go through from beginning to end. Take your time and use a highlighter (I like yellow best) to mark any ideas that stand out. Then go back a few weeks later and start again. See if the same ideas strike you, or perhaps something new will catch your eye and enlighten your mind. Patanjali was the first yogi ever to put the specific instructions for following this path of yoga in writing. Prabhavananda and Isherwood have added commentary that speaks to contemporary needs. It is truly a treasure.

Peace Lagoon

A definite must for a desert island companion. This precious book is a poetic translation of universal wisdom revealed by enlightened beings while they were in their highest meditative consciousness. It contains sacred and powerful prayers recited daily by Sikhs all over the world. Its words are healing and inspiring, they speak to the soul.

Bhagavad Gita

Translation and commentary by Christopher Isherwood & Swami Prabhavananda
This classic not only deserves a place on your bookshelf, but it should be taken off the shelf and read and appreciated. It tells the story of Arjuna, the warrior who did not want to fight and had to be convinced by Lord Krishna (whom he knew simply as his friend), to do his duty and go into battle. The *Bhagavad Gita* (Song of God) details the threefold path of yoga (Tri-Marga): Karma Yoga, Bhakti Yoga, and Gyan Yoga. There are other translations of the *Bhagavad Gita*, but I think this has the best commentary and is easiest to read.

Great Dialogues of Plato *translated by W.H.D. Rouse*

I call your attention to "The Analogy of the Cave," found in Book VII (514A-516B) starting on page 312 of the paperback edition published by Mentor Books in 1956. It is even illustrated with a drawing of the inhabitants of the cave, who represent all of humanity. It shows them dwelling in the dark, unable to see the real world outside the cave, and taking the shadow

294

figures seen on the wall of the cave as their reality. This is one of those classic tales that is so great to read, knowing that its wisdom and truth shall always endure. (You may want to read all of Plato's Dialogues, but this particular one graphically and unforgettably explains the concept of maya, as men mistake the illusion for the reality.)

Autobiography of a Yogi *by Paramahansa Yogananda*

This was one of the first books I ever read about the experiences of a disciple with his spiritual teacher. I couldn't put it down, and stayed up all night reading it for the first time in 1956. Yogananda's adventures, his lessons with his teachers, his eventual move to the United States have made fascinating reading for millions of people.

Avatar *by Jean Adriel*

The author of this book about Meher Baba is an American woman disciple whose experiences at Baba's ashram in India, and the tests he put her through are not only entertaining, but very, very educational. Understanding the relationship of a student to a spiritual teacher is not an easy one for most westerners. It's not built into our culture. Reading such stories can help us understand the concept.

I met Meher Baba in person in 1956 (he died a few years later), when he came to California. In fact, he visited a meditation group that met in my West Hollywood apartment on Wednesday nights. He came with a few of his followers, and gave a "talk" through an interpreter (he was on silence for many years). It was quite an evening.

Of course, the worship of any person, no matter how enlightened he may be, is not the path for me, but there's a lot to be learned from this book in terms of devotion to a spiritual teacher, and how a teacher works with disciples to help them break through the wall of ego.

In Search of the Miraculous *by P.D. Ouspensky*

Ouspensky was, for a period of time, a disciple of the Russian mystic, Gurdjieff. To this day (and I first read it over 40 years ago) I remember some of

295

the exercises in self-awareness from this book. Its main message is that we are all robots, reactive machines without self awareness. It points out that anyone can push our buttons and make us angry, or insecure, etc., until we start to "work on ourselves." The book expounds some very technical, mathematical theories, and I skimmed over those pages, but some of the descriptive material about the types of human behavior is quite interesting. The major flaw, I believe, in Ouspensky's (and/or Gurdjieff's) philosophy, is the emphasis on acquiring personal power without the acknowledgment of God as the real Doer.

"HERE AND NOW" BOOKS AND TAPES

Teachings of Yogi Bhajan *by Yogi Bhajan*

In addition to providing insightful gems of guidance to remember and incorporate in your life, the words in these pages are mantras to be recited. Timeless wisdom by one of the great teachers of the age. Read aloud nine to eleven pages and experience your own inner transformation. "To know wisdom is nothing. To experience wisdom becomes knowledge. Then you can stand through the times."[2] You can enlighten your own consciousness by the power of these spoken words.

The Man Called Siri Singh Sahib

This commemorative volume was produced in 1979 to honor our spiritual Teacher, the Siri Singh Sahib, Bhai Sahib Harbhajan Singh Khalsa Yogiji, on his 50th birthday. It not only contains stories about his life and achievements, but there are wonderful articles that describe the 3HO lifestyle teachings. This book is one of inspiration and education. It outlines the birth and incredible expansion of 3HO in the western hemisphere, and the renaissance of Sikh Dharma that Yogi Bhajan's life and work brought about. It portrays the remarkable success of a remarkable man. His challenge to students: "You should be ten times greater than me!" His admonition: "Don't love me, love my teachings." His philosophy: "It's not the life that matters, it's the courage that you bring to it."[3] His motto: "If you can't see God in all, you can't see God at all."

Don't put this book on the shelf, keep it out where you can read it and reread it and be inspired and reinspired. It's a collector's item.

History of Sikh Dharma of the Western Hemisphere

An awesome panoramic perspective of the spread of the Sikh way of life here in America and Europe from 1969 to 1995. Twenty-five years with the Siri Singh Sahib Bhai Sahib Harbhajan Singh Khalsa Yogiji spearheading the amazing growth and development of western born Sikhs. Beautiful full color photographs enhance this "coffee table" book of history.

YOGIC TECHNOLOGY

"Sadhana Guidelines"

This Manual provides basic information on mudras, mantras and kriyas with many sets of exercises particularly suited to the beginning student. Every Kundalini Yoga student and teacher should have it. Check the Ancient Healing Ways catalog for this and all the other Kundalini Yoga manuals available. Build your library and your expertise.

Psyche of the Golden Shield

(Compiled by Bibiji Inderjit Kaur from the teachings of Yogi Bhajan)

Want to know the right combination of syllables to chant for prosperity, protection, harmony between husband and wife, courage, getting rid of fear, resolving animosity, etc., etc? This is a "handbook of shabds, a celestial energy organizing tool." (A "shabd" is a sound current.) This valuable reference book, contains "Words of prayer, Words of Power, from the Sikh Scriptures that invoke the full power of mantra by reinforcing the psyche in various areas." Translation, transliteration, and the original Gurmukhi script are included.

Psyche of the Soul   *by Siri Singh Sahib Bhai Sahib Harbhajan Singh Khalsa Yogiji & Bhai Sahiba Sardarni Sahiba Bibiji Inderjit Kaur Khalsa*
(Translated and Compiled by Singh Sahib Sant Singh Khalsa, M.D.)

Precious knowledge of the workings of shabd, including the power and promise of the basic daily prayers of the Sikhs (plus others), beautifully translated with Gurmukhi and transliteration. Detailed index. Excellent companion to *Psyche of the Golden Shield.*

297

Furmaan Khalsa *by Siri Singh Sahib Bhai Sahib Harbhajan Singh Khalsa Yogiji*
This beautiful collection of inspired poems is for the serious seeker on the path. A spritual guide for all aspects and facets of life. It is another collector's item, a legacy to give to your children. Originally written by the Siri Singh Sahib, Yogi Bhajan, in Punjabi, the poems have been translated into English by Guruka Singh Khalsa. (Both English and Gurmukhi script are included.)

72 Stories of God, Good and Goods *compiled by Tej Kaur*
A collection of the classic tales of India that have been told by Yogi Bhajan in his lectures throughout the years. A book for adults as well as children.

84 Aspects of Siri Singh Sahib Ji: Life With a Spiritual Teacher
by Wahe Guru Kaur
In this collection of 84 delightful poems, commissioned by the Master of the spoken word himself, Yogi Bhajan, Ph.D., Wahe Guru Kaur has created word pictures of a living master, inspired by seeing him on a day to day basis in a myriad of circumstances and listening to his interaction with people in all walks of life.

Stories to Win the World *by Bibiji Inderjit Kaur*
Stories she was told by her grandparents and has passed along to her children and grandchildren, this wonderful collection gives children the values they need to put in their hearts so that their lives will be noble, successful, and complete as human beings.

HEALING THROUGH FOODS

The Ancient Art of Self-Healing
This is a treasure. From his extensive study and yogic knowledge, Yogi Bhajan gives us information on which specific foods the yogis discovered work on the human body and its ailments: organs, glands, diseases, etc. This is a "must have" reference book. It even has a special section of Foods for Women.

Golden Temple Vegetarian Cookbook *by Yogi Bhajan*

Yes, he's also a master chef! Yogi Bhajan provided many recipes which have been used in the Golden Temple Restaurants throughout the world. Here's a great collection of them for you to try at home.

Conscious Cookery and **From Vegetables With Love** *by Siri Ved Kaur Khalsa*

Two cookbooks from a fabulous cook. Siri Ved Kaur spent several years cooking for Yogi Bhajan personally, under his direction. She learned a lot from him and has produced these marvelous cookbooks, filled with useful and delicious recipes. She even tells where to get the special ingredients for those yogic dishes.

A Taste of India *by Inderjit Kaur*

Known as "Bibiji," Inderjit Kaur is the wife of Yogi Bhajan. Her cooking is the best Indian food I've ever tasted. If you want delicious, authentic recipes from someone who really knows Indian cooking, and also understands western taste, this cookbook is it!

Sugar Blues *by William Dufty*

This book was a revelation for me. It's an exposé, a factual account of the serious damage that refined, white sugar can do to the human body. It even traces the history of the mercenary motives of those who purposely set out to get people hooked on sugar! You may not want to accept the facts in this book, but you owe it to yourself and your children at least to read it. Have you noticed how "hyper" kids get after we give them sugar treats? Ignorance is NOT bliss. Dufty researched for 15 years and concluded that "like opium, morphine, and heroin, sugar is an addictive, destructive drug."

Hypoglycemia, A New Approach *by Dr. Paavo Airola*

I used to eat three candy bars a day to keep my energy up. (Sugar gives energy, right? NOT!) My poor pancreas was working overtime trying to keep my blood sugar level normal. It finally gave up. Hypoglycemia is the opposite end of the spectrum from diabetes. Fortunately, hypoglycemia can be cured

299

through correct diet. If you tend to have major mood swings, are extremely irritable and have a constant craving for sweets, these could be signs of hypoglycemia. This book gives great information as well as some recipes that work wonders in providing solid, satisfying carbohydrates without blowing out your pancreas and adrenals. The author explains why millet and buckwheat are the two best sources of carbohydrate for anyone with hypoglycemia. (They break down into sugar very slowly in the bloodstream, instead of giving you a rush all at once.) The sugar rush caused by many other carbohydrates is like the effect of alcohol in the bloodstream: first comes elation, then the mood plunge into depression, leaving you with an insatiable craving to eat (or drink) more to recapture that "high" again.

Diet for a New America *by John Robbins*
What's Wrong With Eating Meat? *by Barbara Parham*
These books present the case for a vegetarian diet.

NEWSLETTERS

SCIENCE OF KEEPING UP

This is my baby, a newsletter published by the 3HO Foundation. It grew out of my personal correspondence with individual 3HO family members starting in 1969, becoming a general distribution letter when I couldn't keep up with the volume of mail. Then we merged with a newspaper style periodical and called ouselves "Keeping Up Connections." After that came "Still Keeping Up!" and in 1994 it became the "Science of Keeping Up." In this newsletter, to the extent space will allow, I attempt to share as much as possible of Yogi Bhajan's teachings, transcripts of his lectures (excerpts) with commentary by yours truly, as well as sets of exercises and meditations both old and new. You are more than welcome to receive it, simply write to me and ask to be put on the mailing list.

KUNDALINI RISING!

Official newsletter of the International Kundalini Yoga Teachers Association. Please write to IKYTA at 3HO International Headquarters, New Mexico Office, for information about membership at Route 2, Box 4, Shady Lane, Espanola, NM 87532. Phone: (505) 753-5881; FAX (505)753-5982.

PROSPERITY PATHS

A newsletter for and about the Path of Sikh Dharma and Khalsa. Inspiring articles, meditations, lecture transcripts. Contact the Community Development office of Sikh Dharma at Route 2, Box 4, Shady Lane, Espanola, NM 87532 Phone: (505) 753-5881; FAX (505)753-5982.

AUDIO TAPES

With the invention of the auto-reverse tape recorder and the compact disk, we now have the opportunity to use even our sleeping hours to the advantage of our consciousness. This is a short list of a few of my personal favorite tapes. There are hundreds of others to choose from. These can get you started.

NAAD, THE BLESSING by Sangeet Kaur Khalsa singing the *Dhan Dhan Ram Das Guru* shabd. This is the shabd "when you need a miracle." At KWTC, Yogi Bhajan often has this tape played while the campers take a "nap."

NITNEM, THE BANIS recited by Baba Nihal Singh. The sacred daily prayers of the Sikhs. What could be better to put into your subconscious?

JAAP SAHIB Energizing, dynamic words of power. Musical rendition of Guru Gobind Singh's famous hymn in praise of God, sung by renowned Ragi Sat Nam Singh. This tape can be used to help you "keep up" while doing certain Kundalini Yoga Exercises.

GATEWAY TO THE SOUL The daily prayers (banis) recited in English by SS Shanti Shanti Kaur Khalsa, with musical background. (available through Cherdi Kala Music and GT Recordings on audio tape or CD. SS Dr. Sant Singh Khalsa's translation, contents similar to *Peace Lagoon*.)

RAKHE RAKHAN HAR sung by Gurushabd Singh Khalsa. This mantra of protection was composed by Guru Arjan Dev and is recited as part of the Sikh evening prayer, Rehiras.

Here's where you can get these books and tapes:

ANCIENT HEALING WAYS CATALOG
Books,Tapes, Ayurvedic products, Yogi Teas, Essential Oils, Herbs, and much more!
Route 3, Box 259
Espanola, New Mexico, 87532
Phone: (800) 359-2940   (outside USA: (505) 747-2860)
FAX: (505) 747-2868

Golden Temple Enterprises
Audio or Video Tapes of Yogi Bhajan's lectures and classes, current and historic as well as music tapes:
Box 13; Shady Lane
Espanola, NM 87532
Phone: (505) 753-0563   Fax: (505) 753-5603

Cherdi Kala
Audio Music Tapes:
1539 S. Shenandoah St., Apt. #301
Los Angeles, CA. 90035
Phone/Fax: (310) 859-1770

You can also try your local bookstore, or a metaphysical bookstore. If all else fails, write or phone me at 3HO International Headquarters.

INFORMATION

3HO International Headquarters
P.O. Box 351149
Los Angeles, CA 90035
Phone: (310) 552-3416
Fax: (310) 557-8414

International Kundalini Yoga Teachers Association
Route 2, Box 4, Shady Lane
Espanola, New Mexico 87532
Phone: (505) 753-0423
Fax: (505) 753-5982

Yogi Bhajan Home Page
http://www.yogibhajan.com

About the Author

*T*he author was born in Minneapolis, Minnesota, June 19, 1929, the youngest of three children. Her family moved to California in 1942, right after the beginning of World War II. Valedictorian of Hollywood High School, she majored in English at UCLA, with a minor in Psychology, got married, gave birth to a son, was divorced and spent fifteen years exploring various spiritual paths trying to understand what life was all about. After studying with various teachers, she made a pilgrimage to India in 1967.

After her return to Los Angeles, she met Yogi Bhajan at the East West Cultural Center in December of 1968. He told her of his vision of a "Healthy, Happy, Holy Organization" that would train teachers of Kundalini Yoga. He said that her destiny was to be a teacher. Of course, she was skeptical, but the rest, as they say, is history. Since that time, she has devoted her life to practicing and teaching the 3HO way of life, specializing in teaching Kundalini Yoga to beginners. She has traveled to various cities throughout the western hemisphere as a facilitator for Yogi Bhajan's White Tantric Yoga video courses.

Her personal philosophy is, "If you want to be happy, there are two things you have to do (in addition to regular sadhana): have the right containers for everything, and don't take yourself too seriously."

Known as the "Mother of 3HO," Shakti Parwha has been corresponding with the 3HO family since it began, the last few years by producing a Newsletter, "The Science of Keeping Up." It shares the teachings of Yogi Bhajan along with her personal commentary.

Shakti was ordained as a minister of Sikh Dharma in 1974 and is a member of the Khalsa Council, the governing body of the Sikh Dharma of the Western Hemisphere. She is Yogi Bhajan's Executive Secretary, and holds executive offices in both Sikh Dharma and 3HO Foundation.

Glossary

3HO Foundation. Healthy, Happy, Holy Organization

Adi Shakti. Primal Power

Ambrosial Hours. Early morning, 2 1/2 hours before sunrise

Amrit. Nectar of bliss

Apana. Elimination, the eliminating force; the outgoing, cleansing breath of life

Ardas. Prayer (Traditional prayer of the Sikhs)

Asana. Yogic posture, the way to sit

Ascetic. One who lives an austere life of self-denial, renouncing attachment and involvement in worldly activities

Bandh (bandha). Lock

Bhakti Yoga. Yogic path of devotion

Bij Mantra. Seed sound: Sat Nam

Chakras. Energy centers

Dharma. Righteousness

God. Generator, Organizer, and Destroyer (or Deliverer) of all Creation. God is a "Word"

Golden Temple. Most revered and sacred Sikh temple in the world (also called the Harimandir Sahib); located in Amritsar, India; built of marble and gold

Gurbani. Sacred language of the Sikhs, based on Naad, the power inherent in the sound current.

Gurdwara. Sikh temple or place of worship; literally the "gate of the Guru"

Guru. Literally: Gu means darkness; Ru means light: The giver of technology: the teacher. In the Sikh tradition, there were only ten human beings who had the status (consciousness) of "Guru"

Gyan Yoga. Yogic path of the intellect

Hatha Yoga. Yogic path primarily utilizing postures, and emphasizing development of the will

Ida. Left nerve channel (nadi): relates to left nostril, moon energy

Jallunder Bandh. Neck lock

Kama Shastra. Ancient sacred text

Karma. Action and reaction. the cosmic law of cause and effect.

Karma Yoga. Yoga of non-attached action, selfless service in the name of God

Khalsa. Pure one

Kriya. Specific combination of a yogic posture, hand position, breathing, and mantra; literally: a "completed action"

Kundalini. The nerve of the soul; literally "the curl of the lock of hair of the beloved"

Liberation. The experience of your own Infinity

Mahabharata. Epic Vedic writings

Mahan Tantric. Master of White Tantric Yoga; currently Yogi Bhajan

Mantra. Sound current that tunes and controls mental vibration; a syllable or combination of syllables that help focus the mind; words of power; mental vibration to the infinite mind

Maya. Anything which can be measured; usually thought of as the "illusion," i.e., that which we mistake for reality.

Meditation. Letting God talk to you

Mudra. Yogic hand position

Muladhara. The first of the chakras

Naad. Basic sound for all languages through all times originating in the sound current; the universal code behind human communication

Pingala. Right nerve channel (nadi): relates to right nostril; sun energy

Prana. The energy of the atom; essence of life, God's gift to you (that you receive with each inhalation. Breath is the primary carrier of prana.)

Pranayam. Yogic breathing technique

Prasad (prashad). Gift

Prayer. Talking to God

Raj Yoga. Royal path of yoga. Described in Patanjali's aphorisms, translated into *How to Know God. (See recommended reading list)*

Sadhana. Personal spiritual effort on a regular basis

Shabd. Sound; sound current.

Shakti. Woman; God's power in manifestation; feminine aspect of God

Sikh. Literally a seeker of Truth; one who embraces the Sikh religion

Siri Guru Granth Sahib. Living Guru of the Sikhs; a volume containing the sacred words of enlightened beings who spoke or wrote them when they were in a state of union with God (yoga)

Sukhasan. Yogic posture known as "Easy Pose" (usually cross-legged)

Sushumna. Central spinal channel

Tri-Marga. "Three-fold Path" of Karma, Bhakti, and Gyan Yoga described in the *Bhagavad-Gita*

Vedas (vedic texts). Ancient Hindu scriptures; vast body of knowledge, the latter portion of which comprise the Vedanta philosophy

Wahe Guru. Wow! God is great!; mantra of ecstasy expressing the indescribable magnificence of God

Yoga. Union: The science of yoking or uniting the individual consciousness with the Universal consciousness

Yogi . One who has attained a state of yoga, a master of him/her self; person who practices the science of yoga

Chapter Notes

Chapter 1 *What's It All About?*
1 Patanjali was the first yogi to write down the eight steps required to attain mastery following the path of Raj Yoga. A translation with wonderful commentary on his aphorisms was made into a book called *How to Know God* (see Sources & Resources, p.293)
2 November 11, 1991, we entered into twenty-one years of transition into the Aquarian Age, which comes into full force in the year 2013. These twenty-one years are divided into three 7-year periods of increasing intensity.

Chapter 4 *Breath of Life*
1 Genesis.

Chapter 5 *Mantra*
1 Yogi Bhajan.
2 MSS Gurucharan Singh Khalsa Ph.D., "Prosperity Paths," Sikh Dharma Newsletter, 1995.
3 Siri Singh Sahib Yogi Bhajan, Espanola NM Gurdwara lecture, Jan 26, 1992.
4 "The Sacred Science of Kundalini Yoga: The Teachings of Yogi Bhajan, Ph.D." Compiled by Gurucharan Singh Khalsa, Ph.D.
5 "Beneath the rule of men entirely great/ The pen is mightier than the sword." Edward Bulwer Lytton, "Richelieu" Act II, Sc 2 (1839).
6 Excerpt from "Naad Yoga" compiled by MSS Gurucharan S. Khalsa, Ph.D.
7 Excerpt from "The Science of Naad and Gurbani" by Yogi Bhajan.

Chapter 6 *Conquer the Mind, You Conquer the World*
1 Guru Nanak (Manjeet, jagjeet).
2 Yogi Bhajan.

Chapter 7 *Mysterious Kundalini*
1 *Kundalini, Evolution and Enlightenment, Exploring the Myths and Misconceptions*, Edited by John White, Paragon House, 1990, p.144.
2 Swami Prabhavananda and Christopher Isherwood, *How to Know God*, Vedanta Press, 1953, pp. 266-267.
3 *Kundalini, Evolution and Enlightenment: Exploring the Myths and Misconceptions*, p.144
4 *The Teachings of Yogi Bhajan*, p. 177.

307

Chapter 8   *Chakras (Energy Centres) Where Are You At?*
1   Early 3HO song.
2   Kirlian photography used electrical discharges from the skin's surface to see a corona of energy. That corona changed with the emotional states and states of consciousness. It provided a visual analog to the aura and stimulated a lot of research into the connection of body, mind, and spirit. It is not a proven technique, but an interesting experimental procedure.
3   *Kundalini, Evolution and Enlightenment*, p.141. (Best if you read the entire article!)

Chapter 9   *Stress, Stamina & Nerves of Steel*
1   The source of this material is unknown. Someone sent me this story by FAX.

Chapter 10   *Healing*
1   Guru literally means the "Giver of technology." To Sikhs, the word Guru means much more than just teacher, the "Guru" is the embodiment of God. (I'll have to write another book to explain!)

Chapter 13   *Drugs*
1   Yogi Bhajan.
2   Yogi Bhajan.
3   Chaim Weizmann (1874-1952).

Chapter 14   *Sleep*
1   Wm. Shakespeare, "Macbeth," Act II Sc. 1.
    "The death of each day's life, sore labour's bath, Balm of hurt minds,
    Great nature's second cause, Chief nourisher in life's feast."
2   Los Angeles Times, Feb. 10, 1994, "Only Wimps Need 8 Hours."
3   Yogi Bhajan, KWTC.

Chapter 15   *How to Get Up in the Morning*
1   Powdered potassium alum is available for purchase in bulk from Harbhajan Singh: (619) 281-1327 — 2822 Gregory St. San Diego, CA 92104 and in small containers at Yoga West, 1535 S. Robertson Blvd., L.A., CA 90035; (310) 552-4647.
2   From the novel *Fortitude,* by Hugh Walpole, often quoted by Yogi Bhajan.

Chapter 16   *Sadhana: Your Spiritual Bank Account*
1   Yogi Bhajan.
2   Yogi Bhajan.
3   See Sources and Resources for recommendations.

Chapter 17 *Woman is Spelled Double-You-O-Man*
1   Yogi Bhajan, KWTC 1989.
2   Yogi Bhajan, June 24, 1994 (KWTC).
3   From a sacred writing called Asa Di Var in Siri Guru Granth Sahib: p.473 (Manmohan
      translation: p. 1562-3).
4   Yogi Bhajan.
5   Vedic writings, the ending section of which comprise the famous Bhagavad Gita—Song of God.
6   "Power of a Woman" & other excerpts are from Yogi Bhajan's lecture at KWTC, July 8, 1985.

Chapter 20 *Communication*
1   Yogi Bhajan.
2   Copyright: Harbhajan Singh Khalsa Yogiji, 1980.
3   (Exact reproduction on this page of *"The Snake That Poisons Everybody,"* copyright permission
      granted by United Technologies Corporation 1986).

Chapter 22 *Life is a Movie*
1   Guru Nanak, the First Guru of the Sikhs.
2   Part of the song: "One Thing to Remember Is" by Yogi Bhajan.

Chapter 24 *Tantric Yoga*
1   Yogi Bhajan.

Chapter 25 *Ten Bodies*
This chapter contains material reprinted from *A Khalsa Children's Coloring Book*, compiled and
illustrated by Harijot Kaur Khalsa.

Chapter 26 *Going Home*
1   I suggest that you get Yogi Bhajan's lecture tape on this subject and learn more about the
      greatest mystery of life. "Yogi Bhajan speaks on Death and Dying" at the World Parliament
      of Religions Chicago, Illinois, Sept. 4, 1993. Lecture tape #YB174.

THINGS TO DO

How to Chant
1 Yogi Bhajan, KWTC, July 20, 1994.
2 Dhiaan is usually translated simply as "meditation", however Yogi Bhajan elaborated on the concept with the following technical explanation and metaphor: "Dhiaan is locking of the bandas (locks), locking of the chakras (energy centers), and locking of all the tricutes (triangles). In layman's terms, you can understand dharana (usually translated as "concentration"), is "foreplay" (kirtan, simran, japa, naada); Dhiaan is "intercourse," and samadhi is "conception," when the sound and the breath and the self become one.
3 Available from Golden Temple Recordings.
4 Other tapes may be used for meditation, you may chant aloud, or mentally repeat a mantra.
5 Yogi Bhajan, KWTC, July 1994.

Change of Habit Breath Meditation
1 Meditation and commentary as taught by Yogi Bhajan Oct. 22, 1971.

Meditation for Positive Communication
1 Yogi Bhajan: "Communication, Liberation or Condemnation", Page 33; San Francisco, 1980 Reprinted with permission.

Meditation to Clear Past Present Future
1 Yogi Bhajan, KWTC 1993.

Basic Breath Series
1 "Kundalini Yoga Sadhana Guidelines", p. 81.

What's Your Angle?
1 See "Let's talk about Food" Chapter, and the book, *Hypoglycemia, A Better Approach*, by Dr. Paavo Airola.

Sources & Resources
1 Edgar Cayce Research Society has documented thousands of cures based on his teachings.
2 Yogi Bhajan.
3 Based on the opening lines of the novel *Fortitude*, Yogi Bhajan read at the age of nine.

Thanks to 3HO Foundation for permission to use material from *The Science of Keeping Up, Beads of Truth*, and *Women in Training* publications; and to KRI (Kundalini Research Institute) for the use of material from *Sadhana Guidelines*.

Index

Gentle Reader, please note: Topics that have a whole chapter devoted to them, such as Breath or Sleep or Food-Diet-Digestion, have been omitted from this Index, because the Table of Contents will tell you where to find them.